The Fitness Leader's Handbook

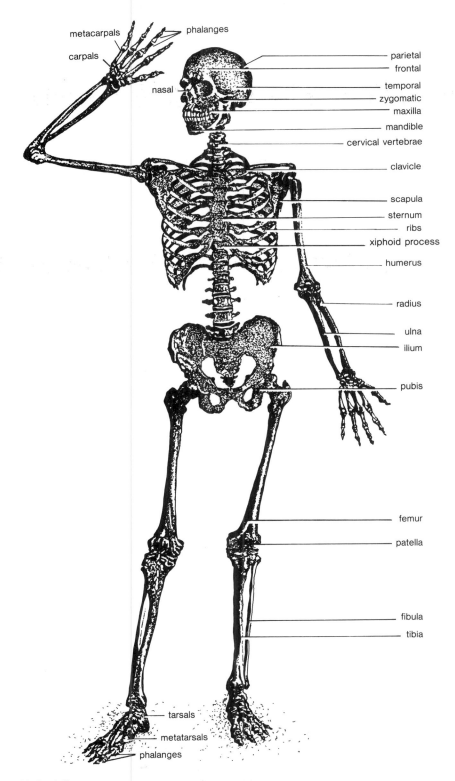

metacarpals

phalanges

carpals

nasal

parietal

frontal

temporal

zygomatic

maxilla

mandible

cervical vertebrae

clavicle

scapula

sternum

ribs

xiphoid process

humerus

radius

ulna

ilium

pubis

femur

patella

fibula

tibia

tarsals

metatarsals

phalanges

Fig. 1.1: The Human Skeletal System

THE FITNESS LEADER'S HANDBOOK

Third Edition

Compiled by
Garry Egger M.P.H., Ph.D. and Nigel Champion B.P.E.

Kangaroo Press

Contributors

Jenny Baker	Occupational Therapist
Lisa Champion	M.Sc., Fitness Consultant. Lecturer, ACHPER Fitness Leader Programs
Nigel Champion	B.P.E., Director, Fitness Leader Network, and Co-ordinator ACHPER Fitness Leader Courses.
Lyn Clark	Aquafitness Instructor, Health Promotion and Media Unit, NSW Department of Health
Bill Daley	B.A., M.Ed., Dip.P.E., Lecturer in Human Movement Studies, Sydney Institute of Education
Garry Egger	B.A.(Hons), M.P.H., Ph.D., Director, Centre for Health Promotion and Research, Sydney, and Fitness Co-ordinator, ACHPER
Carole Renouf	B.A., M.A., Health Promotion Consultant, NSW Department of Health
Rosemary Stanton	B.Sc., C.Nut./Diet., Grad.Dip., Admin., Nutritionist

Our thanks to:

Debbie Tyson for her drawings.
Kathryn Wheatley and Melinda Aldridge for modelling the potentially dangerous exercises.
Margi Payne for modelling

© Garry Egger and Nigel Champion 1983, 1986 and 1990

Reprinted 1991, 1992 and 1993
This third edition published in 1990
First published in 1983 by Kangaroo Press Pty Ltd
3 Whitehall Road (P.O. Box 75) Kenthurst 2156
Typeset by G.T. Setters Pty Limited
Printed by Kyodo Printing Co (S'pore) Pte Ltd

ISBN 0 86417 276 1

Contents

Preface

This handbook has been specifically written for the Fitness Leader Training Programs that are conducted throughout Australia and New Zealand.

The Fitness Leader Program aims to provide all people working, or wishing to work, in the fitness industry with an understanding of the principles for conducting all exercise programs. The program has been specifically designed for fitness instructors, teachers, health professionals and others interested in health and fitness.

The first edition of the Fitness Leader's Handbook was written in 1983. Since then the industry has grown rapidly, not only in size, but also in understanding of scientific exercise principles.

This third edition of the Fitness Leader's Handbook outlines the latest research information on potentially dangerous exercises, succinctly covers the programming principles for weight training, outlines nutritional guidelines (in an easily understandable manner) and a scientific basis for the design of safe and effective exercise programs.

We would like to thank the contributing authors for their expertise and co-operation. We would also like to acknowledge all those fitness leaders who have given us feedback and advice on how to make this book as applicable as possible to the needs of fitness professionals.

Nigel Champion and Garry Egger

1 An Introduction to the Human Body

A knowledge of physical fitness requires a basic understanding of the structure and function of the human body. At the least, this can help develop a respect for the limitations of the body; at most it can aid in planning exercises that are both safe and specific for muscles and joints.

Obviously, such a complex subject can't be covered in a single chapter of a handbook such as this. But it is possible to touch on the basics as they relate to physical activity and exercise.

The Basic Structure of the Body

The basic unit of the body is the cell, which exists in all shapes and sizes. It is within the protoplasm, or jelly-like substance of the cell, that complex biochemical changes occur forming the processes of life as we know it.

Groups of cells combined to perform a similar function are referred to as *tissue*. Examples are nerves, muscles and connective tissue. These in turn form organs and organ systems such as the heart, lungs, stomach, glands, skeleton and epidermis or skin.

Of prime importance to the exerciser are the skeletal system, joints and ligaments, muscles and their attachments, and the cardio-respiratory system.

The Skeletal System

There are 226 bones in the human body, many of which are connected through a variety of joints, allowing movement in multiple directions. The function of these bones is support and movement of the body and storage of red blood cells. Bones not linked by moveable joints (i.e. the skull, the rib cage) provide protection for important internal organs such as the brain and the heart and lungs.

Basically, the skeleton consists of a group of long bones (the arms and legs) for movement, the vertebrae of the back and the bones of the pelvis which provide support, the rib cage and the skull to protect the body's vital organs, and the shorter bundles of bones in the more moveable hands and feet. See Figure 1.1.

Joints are the connections between two or more bones. These can be either fixed (e.g. the ribs) or moveable (e.g. the knee). The moveable joints between bones are those that are used mostly during exercise, and are therefore most prone to misuse, wear and even chronic (gradual) or acute (sudden) injury.

There are five major types of joints, with a basic common structure, shown in Figure 1.2.

The joint cavity between two or more connected bones is surrounded by a *synovial membrane*, within which circulates a jelly-like fluid known as *synovial fluid*. This fluid provides nutrients for the joint surface and helps cushion the impact of the two bones during movement.

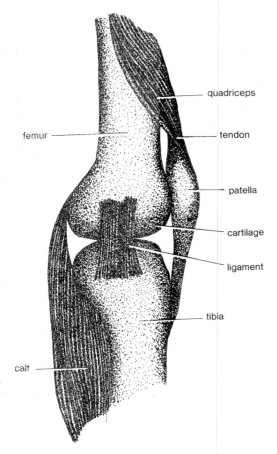

Fig. 1.2: The Structure of a Joint

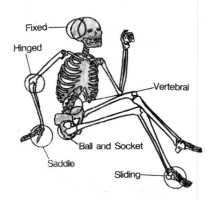

Fig. 1.3: Major Skeletal Joints

Fibrous bands, called *ligaments*, connect the bones on the outside of the synovial membrane, giving the joint stability. However, ligaments are relatively inelastic and respond poorly to sudden dislocation of a joint, often resulting in damage which can last a lifetime. It's imperative therefore that correct exercises

be prescribed for the various joints so that the ligaments are not overstressed but can develop strength and adaptability.

Within the joint itself, the surface of the bones is different in structure to the rest of the bone, being both smoother and less dense. This is called the *articular cartilage*. In addition, some joints (e.g. the knee), have extra pieces of cartilage which help to cushion the impact of the bones. In the knee joint these cartilages are called *menisci*.

Major Skeletal Joints

1. **Ball and socket joints** are so called because the ball-like head of one bone fits into the socket of another, permitting circular movements in most directions. Examples are the shoulder and hip joints.
2. **Hinge joints** open and shut in a similar fashion to a door hinge. Movements that involve narrowing of the angle between joints are called *flexion*, and those involving widening of the angle *extension*. Movement of typical hinge joints, such as the elbow, knee, jaw, fingers and toes, is basically limited to flexion and extension.
3. **Vertebral joints** connect the large bones of the spine. Each individual joint has only limited movement. However, when the vertebrae move together the spine can bend in all directions as well as rotate.
4. **Sliding joints** move from side to side and up and down. They can also rotate, but not as freely as a ball and socket joint. Examples are the wrist and ankle joints, which are also known as *ellipsoid* joints.
5. **Pivot joints** occur where a ring of bone rotates around a bony prominence on another bone. An example is the first cervical vertebra at the base of the skull which rotates around the second cervical vertebra.

The Body as a System of Links

The skeletal system is a system of segments linked together at their joints; thus, the body is called a link system. For exercise instructors, the body is best described by eleven links. These are: the head and neck, the thoracic vertebrae, the lumbar vertebrae, the pelvis, the thigh, the lower leg, the foot, the shoulder girdle, the arm, the forearm, and the hand. The movement of the links in the system takes place at the joints of the segments. Each joint is restricted to movement in one, two or three planes of motion—the sagittal (which divides the body into right and left parts), the frontal (front and back), and the transverse (upper and lower).

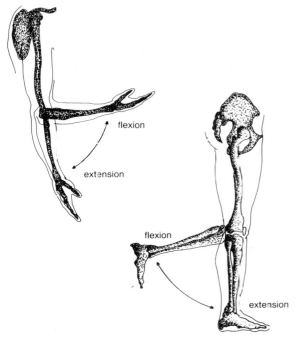

Fig. 1.4: Flexion and Extension a) of the arm
            b) of the leg

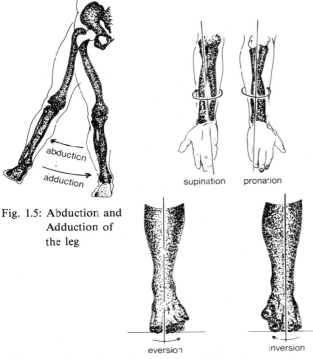

Fig. 1.5: Abduction and
         Adduction of
         the leg

Fig. 1.6: a) Pronation and supranation of the forearm
          b) Eversion and inversion of the foot

Movement Terms

The following terms are commonly used to describe movements of the link system.

Flexion: A movement which makes the angle between two bones at their joint smaller than it was when in the anatomical position. For example, bending the forearm towards the shoulder (see Fig. 1.4).

Extension: Opposite action to flexion. It normally involves lengthening of a muscle or widening of the angle between two bones. For example straightening the arm (see Fig. 1.4).

Abduction: A movement away from the midline of the body. For example moving the arms or legs out to the side (see Fig. 1.5).

Adduction: A movement towards the midline of the body. For example the arms or the legs that are out to the side of the body being brought towards the midline (see Fig. 1.5).

Circumduction: A movement in a circular direction. For example, arm circling is circumduction at the shoulder joint.

Pronation: Where the sole of the foot or hand is turned inward. Often called **inversion**, in relation to the foot (see Fig. 1.6).

Supination: Where the sole of the foot or hand is turned outward. Often called **eversion**, in relation to the foot (see Fig. 1.6).

Plantar flexion: Where the toes are pointed downwards towards the ground (see Fig. 1.7).

Dorsi flexion: Where the toes are pointed upwards towards the knee (see Fig. 1.7).

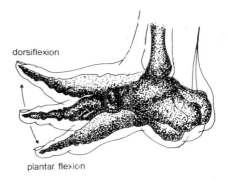

Fig. 1.7: Dorsi and Plantar Flexion

Table 1.1: Muscles and their Functions

Muscle	Origin	Insertion	Action	Bone moved
Biceps	Shoulder and scapula	Radius	Flexion and supination of forearm	Radius and ulna
Triceps	Humerus and scapula	Ulna	Extension of forearm and extension of shoulder	Radius and ulna
Deltoid	Scapula and clavicle	Humerus	Abduction, flexion and extension of shoulder	Humerus
Trapezius	Base of the skull and C7–T12	Clavicle and scapula	Elevation and adduction of scapula	Shoulders
Rhomboids	Spine C7–T5	Scapula	Adduction and downward rotation of scapula	Scapula
Pectorals	Sternum and clavicle	Humerus	Adduction of humerus and flexion	Humerus
Latissimus dorsi	Spine T6–L5	Humerus	Extension, rotation and adduction	Humerus
Rectus abdominus	Pubis	Ribs 5, 6 & 7 Xiphoid process	Trunk flexion	
Erector spinae	Lower 7 ribs to L5 and ilium	C1–L5 and ribs	Back extension	
Gluteals	Ilium and sacrum	Femur	Extension and outward rotation	Femur
Quadriceps— rectus femoris	Ilium	Patella and tibia	Hip flexion and lower leg extension	Femur, tibia and fibula
Hamstrings	Ischium	Tibia	Hip extension and lower leg flexion	Femur, tibia and fibula
Gastrocnemius	Femur	Achilles calcaneus	Knee flexion Plantar flexion	Foot
Soleus	Tibia and fibula	Achilles calcaneus	Plantar flexion	Foot
Tibialis anterior	Tibia	Ankle	Dorsi flexion	Foot

The Muscular System

Approximately 40% of body mass is made up of muscle tissue, the purpose of much of which is to move bones. There are three different types of muscle: smooth muscle (e.g. arteries, stomach), cardiac muscle (e.g. the muscles of the heart) and striated muscle (e.g. arms, legs, etc.). The first two are primarily concerned with involuntary actions. Striated or skeletal muscle, so named because of its striped appearance, generally performs voluntary movements.

There are over 400 muscles in the body but those of major importance to the fitness leader are shown in Figures 1.8 and 1.9.

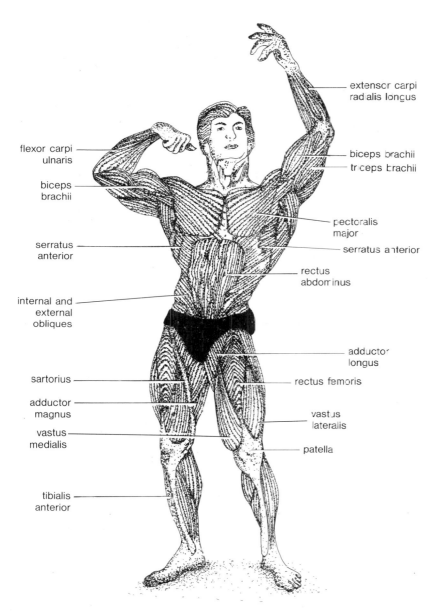

Fig. 1.8: The Muscular System: front view

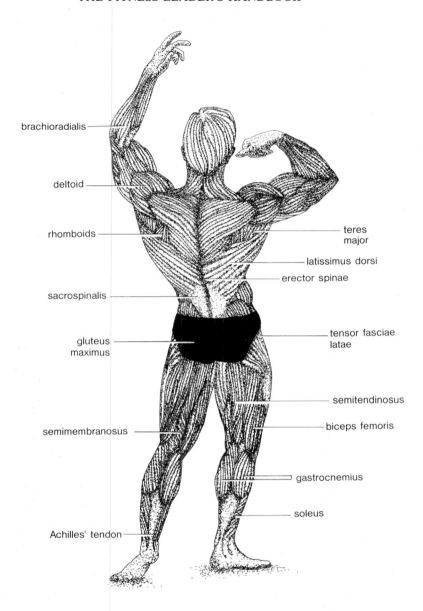

brachioradialis

deltoid

rhomboids

sacrospinalis

gluteus
maximus

semimembranosus

Achilles' tendon

teres
major

latissimus dorsi

erector spinae

tensor fasciae
latae

semitendinosus

biceps femoris

gastrocnemius

soleus

Fig. 1.9: The Muscular System: back view

There are two important factors that the fitness instructor should consider when studying skeletal muscles for exercise prescription purposes:

1. Skeletal muscles only pull on a bone they do not push a bone.

2. Skeletal muscles usually work in pairs. So, consideration should always be given to training the agonist as well as the antagonist or opposing muscle or muscle group.

Muscles Only Pull They Do Not Push

The primary action of skeletal muscles is pulling. *Muscles do not push.* An example is the bicep muscle which pulls the forearm to the shoulder. The bicep plays no role in straightening the arm. It is the tricep muscle that pulls the arm so that it is straightened to an extended position.

This may appear very simple at first but when gravity comes into play the whole process becomes more complicated. Take for example the bicep curl exercise. In the upward movement the biceps are shortening while they are contracting (this is known as a concentric or positive contraction) to bring the bar towards the shoulder. As the weight is lowered (the arms are now straightening) the biceps are working against gravity and act as a braking mechanism. They do this by contracting while the muscle fibres are lengthening (this is known as an eccentric or negative contraction).

Another example is the push-up. Here, the muscles being worked are the pectorals, the deltoids (anterior) and the triceps. When the body is lowered to the floor the triceps are working eccentrically and when the arms are extended to push up from the floor the triceps are working concentrically. The biceps have no role in the push-up exercise.

Always Train the Opposing Muscle or Muscle Group

Muscle balance is often a forgotten element in program prescription, whether it be planning an aerobic track or writing a resistance training program. Many of the skeletal muscles work in pairs and if one muscle is overworked at the expense of the opposing muscle it may predispose the area to injury. A common example of this is anterior lower leg pain which is often referred to as 'shin splints'. This complaint can often be attributed to an imbalance between the strong calf muscles (gastrocnemius and soleus) and the weaker muscle in the shin (tibialis anterior). In a floor class the calf muscles tend to be excessively overloaded due to the amount of jumping exercises and the repetitive foot strike movements that are part of many aerobic

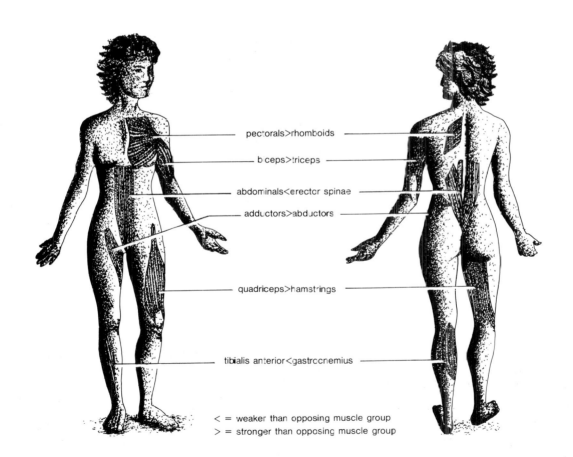

pectorals>rhomboids

biceps>triceps

abdominals<erector spinae

adductors>abductors

quadriceps>hamstrings

tibialis anterior<gastrocnemius

< = weaker than opposing muscle group
> = stronger than opposing muscle group

Fig. 1.10: Muscle Balance (Redrawn from 'Dance Exercise Today', 1988 student handout)

tracks. The calf muscles can become over developed and tighten, thereby creating an imbalance with the weaker tibialis anterior muscle. Figure 1.10 lists those muscles that fitness instructors should consider in order to prevent muscle imbalance.

The Origin and Insertion of Skeletal Muscles

Each skeletal muscle (i.e. that attached to a bone or bones) has an *origin* and an *insertion* and the location of these determines the direction in which it moves a particular bone.

The origin of a muscle is usually the fixed end or the end which does not move during muscle contraction. The insertion is usually the attachment at the bone that is moved by the muscle. (See Figure 1.11.)

Where a muscle approaches its attachment site with a bone, the contractile elements of that muscle end and connective tissue known as *tendons* form the attachment. Some of the fibres (called *collagen fibres*) join with the outside layer of the bone (the *periosteum*) to form a unit which gives strong resistance to any force against the muscle.

Muscles can either contract (shorten) or relax (lengthen). To move a bone, one or more muscles (called the *agonists*) contract, while others (called the *antagonists*) relax, to facilitate the movement. Effective movement of a part of the body therefore depends both on the strength of the *agonist*, and effective co-ordination with the *antagonist*.

The prescription of exercise is highly dependent on the structure and function of the muscle being exercised, and the purpose for which it is being exercised (i.e. strength, flexibility, endurance). A knowledge of the origins and insertions of a muscle can give an indication of whether a specific exercise is having the desired effect on a particular muscle.

For example, the traditional method of teaching sit-ups was to instruct the exerciser to keep his or her legs straight, often by hooking the toes under a fixed attachment. However, in this position two groups of muscles come into play—the abdominals (the desired muscle group), and a muscle called the iliopsoas. This muscle has its origin in the bones of the pelvis and spine, and its insertion in the femur (see Figure 1.12). Because of its connection to the spine, it's thought that if this muscle is selectively over-strengthened, it will cause strain on the lower spine. In any case, it's not the desired muscle for development.

From a knowledge of origins and insertions, it can

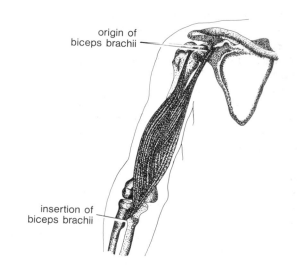

Fig. 1.11: The Origin and Insertion of Biceps Brachii

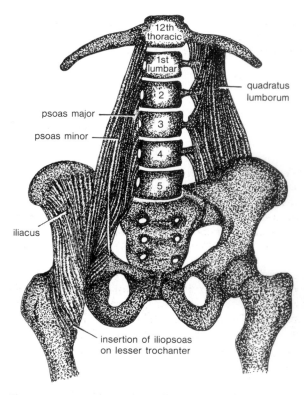

Fig. 1.12: Connections of the Iliopsoas Muscle

be reasoned that if the femur is brought towards the spine (i.e. the leg is bent at the hip), movement of the iliopsoas muscle will be restricted. Bending the knees to perform sit-ups then reduces the involvement of the deeper iliopsoas, and increases the involvement of the abdominals. Hence abdominal strengthening through sit-ups should always be carried out with legs bent.

A second example comes from exercises designed to stretch the muscles of the calf. There are two major muscles of interest here; the *gastrocnemius* or large calf muscle, and the *soleus*, or deeper calf muscle.

When stretching the calf, as is often advisable before and after activity involving the lower limbs, there are two options. The stretch can be carried out with the leg either straight or bent. With the leg straight, both the soleus and gastrocnemius are stretched. With the leg bent, however, there is no stretching of the gastrocnemius because its origin is above the knee joint. With the knee bent, the distance between its origin and insertion has been shortened to less than the length at which stretching takes place (see Figure 1.13). The soleus on the other hand, is stretched much more effectively with the leg bent than with it straight because a greater angle can be achieved at the ankle joint with a bent leg. Since this is the only joint over which the soleus passes—its insertion being below the knee—stretching is maximised through bending.

More detail of muscle physiology in relation to exercise will be covered in Chapter 2.

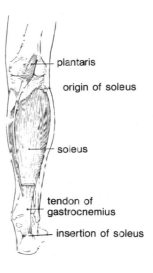

Fig. 1.13: Soleus Muscle (shown with overlying gastrocnemius removed)

The Cardiorespiratory System

The cardiorespiratory system consists of the cardio-vascular system (the heart and blood vessels) and the respiratory system (lungs and air passages). Together, both systems work to transport oxygen to the cells of the working muscles and organs and to remove carbon dioxide and other waste products.

Blood is the fluid that flows through the circulatory system. Approximately 45% of blood volume is composed of red and white blood cells and blood platelets. The remainder is *plasma* which carries food, minerals, hormones and chemical substances needed for life. Red blood cells are able to transport and give up oxygen and carbon dioxide through iron-protein molecules called *haemoglobin*.

The circulatory system consists of **arteries** and **veins**. The former are more elastic than the latter and transport oxygen-rich blood away from the heart. Through poor nutrition, inactivity and other lifestyle factors (e.g. smoking), the arteries can become less elastic and less efficient in blood transport, resulting in excessive strain on the heart or blood pump.

Blood pressure is a measure of the force the heart needs to push blood through the body. It shows the resistance of the blood vessels to the flow of blood around the circulatory system. There are two recordings of blood pressure taken; the first is *systolic blood pressure* and the second is *diastolic blood pressure*.

Systolic pressure is the pressure on the artery walls when the heart contracts and pumps blood through the body. Diastolic pressure is the pressure in the artery walls between pumps or heart beats, when the heart is relaxing.

The Lungs

The lungs (see Figure 1.14) are the organs used to exchange air between the blood and the external environment. Air passes from the environment to the *trachea* or wind passage and through to the *bronchi*, which divide into the two lungs. Within each lung, each bronchus divides and subdivides ending in air sacs called *alveoli*. It is the alveoli which effect the passage of oxygen into and carbon dioxide out of the blood stream.

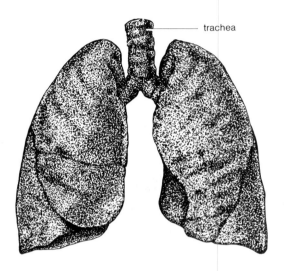

Fig. 1.14: The lungs exchange air between blood and external environment

At rest, the lungs breathe in about 6 to 8 litres of air per minute. However, this amount increases on exertion resulting in more needed oxygen being supplied ultimately to the working muscles.

The Heart

The heart is a muscle which acts as a pump to pump blood through the body. It does this at a rate of approximately 72 beats per minute in the average middle-aged male (80 b.p.m. for females), each beat being called a *pulse*.

The heart, lungs, muscles and organs are connected by veins and arteries that pump blood in a cycle around the body, returning for replenishing and disposal of wastes (see Figure 1.15).

The fact that the heart is called upon to supply more blood to an exercising muscle than a resting muscle is important to the fitness leader, because it means that *pulse rates* can be used as a means of determining the individual's response to exercise and an exercise programme can be planned accordingly. The workings of the heart and the use of pulse rates will be considered in more detail in Chapters 2 and 4.

Major Problems of the Cardiovascular System

Heart Attack

A heart attack (myocardial infarction) results when an artery carrying blood to the heart muscle (coronary artery) becomes blocked (see Figure 1.16). This generally occurs in the presence of partial blockage caused by a disease called *atheroma*.

Atheroma is a build up of fats (cholesterol in particular) and fibrous material on the lining of the arteries. This build-up is gradual and takes place over a person's lifetime. When complete blockage occurs, and this is usually a sudden event, a part of the heart muscle loses its blood supply and dies, hence the term *myocardial* (heart muscle) *infarction* (death of tissue).

Valvular Disease

The heart has valves which allow blood to flow in one direction but not the other. If these valves become damaged, as they may do from various diseases, the normal passage of blood flow is interrupted. The

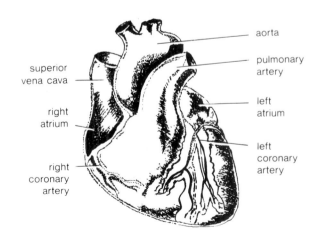

Fig. 1.16: Atheroma and Heart Attack

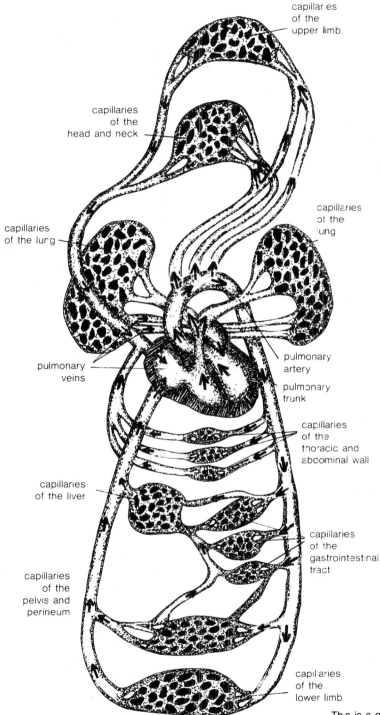

capillaries of the upper limb

capillaries of the head and neck

capillaries of the lung

capillaries of the lung

pulmonary veins

pulmonary artery

pulmonary trunk

capillaries of the thoracic and abdominal wall

capillaries of the liver

capillaries of the gastrointestinal tract

capillaries of the pelvis and perineum

capillaries of the lower limb

This is a generalised diagram of the body circulation plan and is not anatomically accurate. Use it to see how blood leaves the heart, reaches a body region, distributes nutrients/gases at the capillary level and returns to the heart.

Fig. 1.15: Schematic Diagram of the Circulatory System

damage can often be detected by a heart murmur or 'whooshing' sound which is audible through a stethoscope.

Disturbances of Rhythm

Under some circumstances the heart may beat irregularly (and therefore inefficiently). There are a variety of causes, and all require detailed medical inspection.

Pooling of Blood

There are some situations where pooling of blood may occur in the venous system, particularly in people who may have to stand for long periods during hot weather. This means simply, that blood is not returned to the heart and lungs for re-oxygenating and delivery to the muscles and organs of the body, including the brain. Fainting can result, leading to a correction of the problem because it removes the gravitational effect contributing to the pooling of blood.

Anatomical Positions

The following are terms commonly used to describe locations in body structure:

Superior: Towards the head, or 'upper' or 'above'.
Inferior: Towards the feet, or 'lower' or 'below'.
Anterior: Front or 'in front of'.
Posterior: Back or 'at the back of'.
Medial: Towards the midline of the body.
Lateral: Towards the side of the body.
Proximal: Towards or nearest the trunk of the body or nearest the point of origin of a body part.
Distal: Away from or farthest from the trunk or the point of origin of a body part.

Dorsal: Also used to describe back or 'posterior'.
Ventral: Also used to describe front or 'anterior'.
Sagittal: A sagittal plane is a lengthwise plane running from front to back, i.e. it divides the body into right and left.
Frontal: A frontal plane divides the body into anterior and posterior sections.
Transverse: A transverse plane is a horizontal or crosswise plane dividing the body into upper and lower sections.
Supine: Lying face upwards.
Prone: Lying face downwards.

2 The Human Body and Exercise

For the human body to function, it needs energy. Energy for activity is provided in the muscles in the form of an energy rich molecule known as *adenosine triphosphate* (ATP), which is the basic energy currency for muscle contraction. Millions of ATP molecules are stored in the muscle. In order for the muscle cell to contract, ATP molecules are broken down to ADP (adenosine diphosphate) and energy is released (Fig. 2.1). In order for the muscle to continue to contract the ADP must be rebuilt back to ATP. There are a number of processes by which this occurs and these will be explained in this chapter.

Two forms of energy concern us here—mechanical and chemical. *Chemical energy* in the body is the result of the breakdown of foodstuffs, some of which is converted into energy compounds. These are then broken down and used by the skeletal muscles in performing *mechanical work*.

The most common unit of measure of energy is the calorie (now replaced by the kilojoule; 1 calorie = 4.2 joules). A *calorie* is the amount of heat energy required to raise the temperature of 1 gram of water 1 degree centigrade. A *kilocalorie* (kcal) is equal to 1000 calories and is the unit most often used in describing the energy content of foods and the energy requirements of various physical activities.

For example, one 280 gram glass of beer would contain around 100 calories (429kJ). In exercise terms, this would be roughly equivalent to running a mile in 6 minutes 30 seconds. Around 3800 calories (16,250kJ) amount to 0.5kg of body fat, which unless burned as energy is stored as *adipose* (fat) tissue in the body.

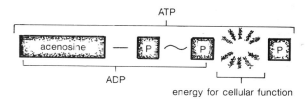

$ATP \rightarrow ADP$ + Energy for biological work + P
(ADP = adenosine diphosphate)

Fig. 2.1: The ATP Molecule

The Energy Systems

All human movements require energy. But the method by which the body generates energy (i.e. reproduces ATP as it is used up in the muscles) is determined by the intensity and duration of an activity. Activities that require sudden bursts of effort such as jumping and sprinting need a large production of energy over a short period of time. At the other extreme, activities like distance running and cycling are mostly low power output activities that call for continued energy production over a prolonged period.

The first of these types of movement (sudden bursts) are powered by energy systems that don't require oxygen. They're termed *anaerobic*, which literally means 'without air'. In these cases, energy comes from high energy phosphate substances in the muscle (the phosphate energy system) or from the use of sugar materials in the muscle, resulting in the production of lactic acid (the lactate energy system).

More extended activities like jogging and cycling require a supply of oxygen to produce continued activation of muscles. Hence these are called *aerobic* (with air) activities. Figure 2.2 shows the relationship between the various energy systems.

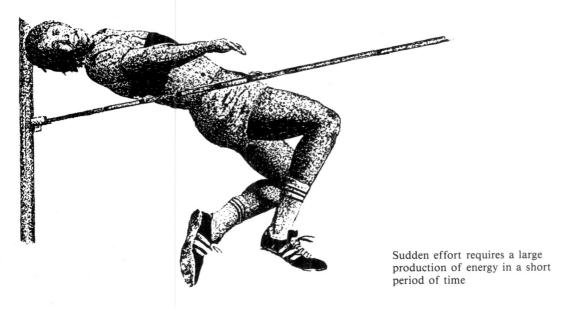

Sudden effort requires a large production of energy in a short period of time

The Aerobic System

The aerobic system is perhaps the most important energy pathway for active individuals to understand because it is the system the body uses for everyday living. It's also the system that predominates in long distance events. In fact, the marathon event is often considered to be a pure aerobic event.

The aerobic system is so called because it is energy produced in the presence of air, or oxygen. During vigorous activity, the exercising muscles use increasing amounts of oxygen and produce carbon dioxide and water as by-products.

As the efficiency of the cardiovascular system in carrying oxygen to the muscles improves (i.e. through improved fitness), the total amount of oxygen consumed by the working muscles per minute increases. The maximal value, often expressed in terms of millilitres of oxygen per kilogram of bodyweight per minute (ml/kg/min) is called an individual's *aerobic capacity* or *maximal oxygen uptake (MVO$_2$)*. Theoretically, a higher MVO$_2$ indicates an increased ability of the heart to pump blood to the lungs to ventilate oxygen and of the muscles to take up oxygen.

The series of reactions producing energy via the aerobic system takes place within the muscle cells. But they are confined to specialised sub-cellular sections of muscle tissue called *mitochondria*. These are often referred to as the 'powerhouses' of the cell because of their role in the aerobic manufacture of ATP energy.

Aerobic energy requires the use of carbohydrates and fats. These are broken down, through a process of some 20–25 chemical steps to form ATP, with water and carbon dioxide as by-products (see Table 2.1). The water formed is useful within the cell itself and the carbon dioxide is exhaled through the respiratory process. Unlike the anaerobic system, the aerobic system is capable of producing large amounts of ATP without simultaneously generating fatiguing by-products. Basically, activities that utilise aerobic metabolism are those which:

1. Increase the heart rate (i.e. to >120 beats per minute).
2. Use the large muscles of the body (thighs, trunk, arms and shoulders).
3. Are carried out over an extended period (minimum of 15–20 minutes).

These activities include walking, swimming, jogging, cross-country skiing, dancing, cycling, rowing, skipping, circuit training, etc.

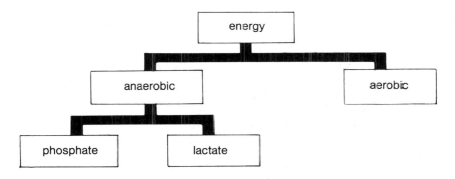

Fig. 2.2: The Energy Systems

The Anaerobic System

Anaerobic energy is simply a way of producing energy without depending on oxygen. This comes into play when the intensity of an activity increases to a point where the cardiorespiratory system can't supply sufficient oxygen to meet the body's energy demands.

Anaerobic energy use is like taking money from a bank. You can't continue to withdraw without making a deposit. In the same way, an oxygen debt is quickly built up from anaerobic activity which must eventually be replaced: the sprinter has to stop and catch his breath; the footballer has to slow down and jog between explosive sprints.

Within the anaerobic system, there are two distinctly different methods of producing energy: the *lactate system* and the *phosphate system*. The former is a means of supplying instant energy through food sources in the absence of oxygen, and the latter comes from the muscles' energy reservoir for instant energy.

the absence of oxygen, this results in the formation of a waste product known as **lactic acid** (see Table 2.1).

If the intensity of the activity is maintained, lactic acid will accumulate in the muscles and blood, resulting in muscle fatigue. Fatigue will start at around 35–40 seconds of vigorous activity, and exhaustion will occur after about 55–60 seconds. Once lactic acid is produced, it requires 45–50 minutes to be removed from the system, and for the individual to recover.

The lactate system is extremely important as it provides a rapid supply of ATP energy for intense, short bursts of activity. It also acts as an energy reserve for the middle or long distance runner to 'kick' in the sprint finish, or for the footballer to accelerate instantly to beat an opponent. Sprinting up to 400 metres makes use predominantly of the lactate system. Middle distance running on the other hand uses predominantly aerobic energy.

The Lactate System

Under circumstances of sprint-like effort, glycogen in the muscles is broken down to form *pyruvic acid* and then ATP energy to replace that burned up in the muscles. This process is called *glycolosis* and it represents only about 5% of the number of ATPs that are produced when glycogen is completely broken down in the presence of oxygen (i.e. aerobically). It is therefore a less efficient means of energy use than aerobic energy.

Also, as glycogen is only partially broken down in

The Phosphate System

The third process for supplying energy to the muscles is the phosphate system. This comes into play when there is insufficient time for the body to break down glycogen for the manufacture of ATP energy. Although ATP serves as the energy currency for all cells, its quantity is limited and only about 85 grams would be stored in the body at any one time. Thus ATP must be constantly resynthesised to provide a continuous supply of energy.

For brief, dynamic bursts of energy (e.g. lifting a heavy weight), the ATP already stored in the muscle cells combines with *phosphocreatine*, another high

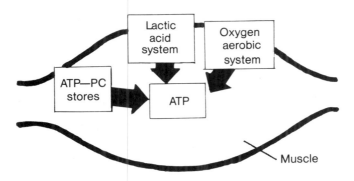

Fig. 2.3: The 3 Systems of Energy Supply to Skeletal Muscle (From Fox, E., 1979)

energy substance which is stored in the muscle. This provides enough energy for 5–10 seconds of maximal effort (see Table 2.1).

As rapidly as these energy supplies are broken down, they are restored, to the extent that 50% of the energy source is available 30 seconds later, and 100% within 2 minutes. As a result, it's possible to repeat many intense but short bouts of activity without becoming exhausted.

In almost all sports, the phosphate system plays a role for short intense bursts of activity. However, if the all-out effort has to continue for longer than about 8 seconds, an additional source of energy must be provided for the resynthesis of ATP. This comes from the food sources which are used or stored for later use to provide the energy to recharge the supply of ATP and PC.

Table 2.1: Energy for Muscle Contraction

	Energy for muscle contraction		
	Anaerobic system (No O_2)		**Aerobic system (with O_2)**
	Phosphate (ATP–PC)	**Lactic**	
Intensity of effort	Very high intensity 95–100% of max effort Explosive	High intensity 60%–95% of max effort	Low intensity Up to 60% of max effort
Duration	Only lasts for 10 seconds of explosive activity	If working at: 95% about 30 seconds 60% about 30 minutes	At low intensity there is no limit
Fuel	Phosphocreatine (PC)	Carbohydrate *only* In the form of: 1. muscle glycogen 2. blood sugar	1. Carbohydrates 2. Fat 3. Protein
Waste product	No waste product	Lactic acid (the incomplete breakdown of carbohydrates)	Carbon dioxide (CO_2)—we breathe it out Water (H_2O)—sweat or pass it out
Recovery time	Very quick 50%—30 seconds 100%—2 minutes	It takes 20 minutes to 2 hours to break down the lactic acid	Time to replace fuel stores

The Relationship between Aerobic and Anaerobic Energy

Short sprints and sudden bursts of activity are generally anaerobic. High performance athletic feats are anaerobic but require an aerobic base. General programs for the development of cardiovascular fitness, on the other hand, do not require anaerobic development but should rely primarily on aerobic activities.

Most activities and sports call on energy from a combination of the aerobic and anaerobic systems (see Table 2.2).

Table 2.2: Examples of different activities and the proportional energy contribution of each energy source

Activity	Duration	Major energy source(s)
Single movement	1 sec.	phosphate
Short sprint	10 sec.	phosphate
Sustained sprint	10–60 secs	phosphate/lactate
Middle distance sprint	1–6 min.	lactate/aerobic
Marathon	2 hrs+	aerobic
Team games/ extended circuit training, floor classes etc.	1 hr+	phosphate/lactate/ aerobic

An intermediate exercise to music class utilises a combination of the aerobic and anaerobic energy systems. As such, it is technically incorrect to refer to it simply as an aerobic class. Take for example a single peak intermediate class where the first 25 minutes involves numerous travelling and high/low impact moves. The large muscles of the legs are being predominantly used, requiring a large blood supply. As a result there is an increase in heart rate which stays elevated for 20 to 25 minutes thereby overloading the aerobic system. There will be times during this part of the class where the intensity is too great for the aerobic system, resulting in oxygen debt and the subsequent accumulation of lactic acid. In addition the anaerobic (phosphate) pathway may be brought into play during high impact moves that require explosive muscle contractions.

The second part of a single peak class is structured to overload different muscle groups. Heart rate drops quite significantly as all movements are done more slowly and in a controlled manner. The anaerobic (lactic) pathway becomes the predominant system in this part of the class. Care should be taken to overload the muscles but not to 'burn' them out completely.

A newcomer to any extended exercise program, such as a floor class, or jogging or swimming, would tire

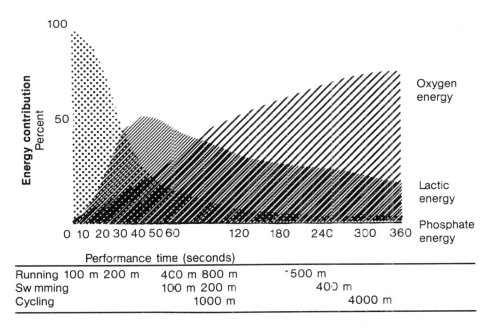

Fig. 2.4: Contribution of Energy Systems to Sports Events (modified from Pyke & Watson, 1978)

quickly because the aerobic system wouldn't be able to cope with the energy demands placed on it. To overcome this, the body calls on anaerobic sources. But this causes tiredness because of the build-up of lactic acid. As the individual adapts to the exercise routine, the aerobic system becomes more efficient, hence muscles don't have to rely as much on anaerobic sources of energy. In lay terms, this means the individual is getting 'fitter'.

The Energy Systems While Out for a Run

Another way of looking at the energy continuum is to imagine you are out on a 6 kilometre comfortable run. Muscle energy for basic metabolism while jogging along at a comfortable pace comes from the aerobic pathway. Now let's consider when and why the other energy systems may come into play during the run.

1. While jogging along you come to a reasonably steep hill and you have two choices. The first choice is to slow down and walk up the hill thereby reducing the intensity, which will ensure that you continue to work aerobically. The second choice is to run up the hill at the same speed as when you were running along the flat. If you do this, the intensity of the run is going to be increased significantly. Your heart will have problems supplying the working muscles with the required increase in oxygen, thereby placing you in 'oxygen debt' and causing you to breathe more heavily. In order to service this increase in energy demand your

muscles start to work anaerobically (in the absence of oxygen) and produce the waste product lactic acid. If the hill is really steep and long you will get into severe oxygen debt and produce large amounts of lactic acid. You may reach a point where your legs start to feel very 'rubbery' and you will have to consider slowing down and maybe even walking. On reaching the top of the hill you cruise down the other side. The heart can easily handle this reduced workload and you start to work aerobically again. The lactic acid is removed from the muscle and broken down by a complex chemical procedure. You are no longer in oxygen debt and can get back to enjoying your run and preparing for the next hill.

2. You have fully recovered from the hill and you are enjoying the scenery when a dog suddenly jumps out of a driveway and starts to chase you. You sprint down the road for 50 metres until the dog loses interest. The energy for this sudden explosive sprint comes from the high energy phosphate stores in your muscles. You only have 10 seconds worth of these stored phosphates so if the dog had kept chasing, you might have been in a bit of trouble! With the threat of the dog left behind you overcome your oxygen debt and slot back into your aerobic system and start to enjoy the scenery again.

Hence, although the ultimate energy currency of muscle contraction is in the form of ATP for jogging along the flat, running up the hill and sprinting from the dog, the means by which it is broken down and reproduced differs according to the type of activity carried out.

The Fuel for Exercise

ATP is made available from food—carbohydrates, proteins and fats. As we have seen, the process by which this occurs can be either aerobic or anaerobic.

Carbohydrate as a Fuel

The most immediate source of fuel comes from carbohydrates which are basically sugars and starches.

Sugars are the simplest form of carbohydrate. Single unit sugars, known as monosaccharides are glucose, fructose and galactose. Double sugars or disaccharides

are sucrose, lactose and maltose. Sugars tend to be labelled as bad—but in fact they are an important part of the diet. It is the processed sugars that have had all nutritional value removed that should be deemed bad.

Starches are complex carbohydrates known as polysaccharides. They are made up of many units of monosaccharides and are found mainly in cereals, grains, vegetables and legumes.

All regularly exercising people should have a diet high in starch and supplemented with sugar. Carbohydrate fuel is stored in the body's cells in two usable forms—glucose and glycogen.

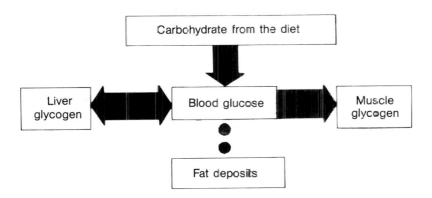

Fig. 2.5: The Relationship between Carbohydrate, Glycogen and Fat Deposits

Glucose (often referred to as blood sugar) is the basic usable form of carbohydrate in the body. Blood sugar levels are important to the normal functioning of the body as it is the only fuel that the brain uses. If blood sugar levels are low (hypoglycemia) lethargy sets in as the whole system starts to slow down. As the name suggests, blood glucose is transported around the body in the blood. In the muscle the blood glucose is stored in the fibres as muscle glycogen (a number of glucose molecules linked together). Glycogen is also stored in the liver which tends to act as the body's reserve tank for carbohydrate. If the body's glycogen stores are full, the glucose is converted and stored as fat (see Figure 2.5).

When glycogen is broken down aerobically, it's broken down completely, with the waste products being water and CO_2. When it's broken down anaerobically on the other hand it's only partially broken down, resulting in the accumulation of lactic acid.

Fat as a Fuel

Like carbohydrate, fat has a basic usable form in the body as free fatty acids (FFA). *Triglycerides* are the FFAs stored in the adipose (fat) tissue and in the skeletal muscles. The mobilisation of FFA from the fat stores to the muscles is important in the control of body weight, because during prolonged exercise of moderate intensity, FFA represent the major source of fuel for ATP production. Furthermore, FFA can *only* be mobilised as an energy fuel via the aerobic system.

In practical terms, this means that stored fats are most readily used as fuel at either low levels of exercise intensity (i.e. slow walking, jogging etc.), or after the body's glycogen supplies have been depleted. Therefore, for decreasing fat on an overweight individual, the early stages of an exercise program can more profitably be structured around gentle, rhythmic exercise rather than around exercises of high intensity.

Muscle Physiology

The component of a muscle cell that distinguishes it from all other cells is the *myofibril*. Skeletal muscle is composed of thousands of these myofibrils bound together by connective tissue and contained in a fluid called *sarcoplasm* (see Figure 2.6).

A myofibril contains two basic protein filaments, a thicker one called *myosin* and a thinner one called *actin*. It is the arrangement of these filaments which gives a muscle its striped or striated appearance, and it's also the movement of these filaments sliding across each other which causes the muscle to contract (see Figure 2.7).

The actual mechanism involved in the sliding process is not fully understood. But the suggested process and the connection with ATP production is summarised in the following series of steps:

Stage	Muscle Action
1. Rest	Cross bridges extended towards actin. Actin and myosin in uncoupled position.
2. Stimulation	Ca++ released. Actin and myosin = actomysin.

3. Contraction   Cross bridges swivel or collapse. Muscle shortens; actin slides over myosin. Tension developed
ATP = ADP + Pi + energy.

4. Relaxation   Stimulation ceases. Ca+ + removed. Muscle returns to resting state.

Nerves and Muscular Movement

Muscular movement is possible through the stimulation of a muscle (the motor nerve) and feedback on the outcome of that movement (the sensory nerve).

The Motor Unit

The function of the motor nerve is to stimulate the muscle fibres so that they will contract. One motor nerve can divide into numerous smaller nerves and service as many as 200 muscle fibres. An individual motor nerve fibre plus all the muscle fibres it innervates is called a *motor unit*.

An increase in the strength of a muscle can be attributed as much to the recruitment of muscle fibres as to the size of the muscle fibres. For example, if the motor units in the bicep brachii muscle fire intermittently when doing a bicep curl the force exerted on the bar is going to be small. If on the other hand all the motor nerves fire in unison then the recruitment of muscle fibres will be greater, resulting in a stronger contraction. Recruitment of muscle fibres is based on training and the muscle is literally taught to contract through each specific movement.

The Sensory Nerves

The function of the sensory nerves (proprioceptors) is to relay back information concerning the muscles, tendons, ligaments and joints. The primary purpose of the proprioceptive system is to make us aware of limb positions and movements, kinesthetic awareness.

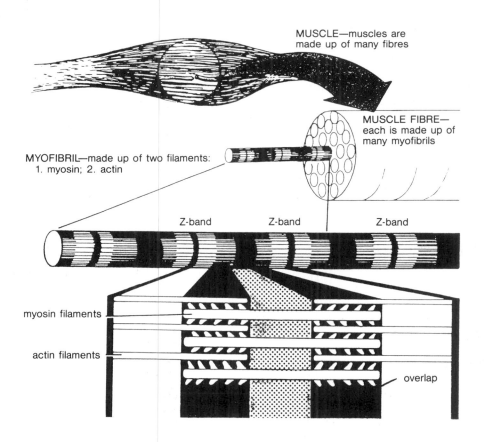

Fig. 2.6: The Basic Structure of Muscle Tissue

There are three important proprioceptors that are concerned with kinesthesis: muscle spindles, Golgi tendon organs and joint receptors.

Muscle Spindles

Muscle spindles send information to the central nervous system concerning the degree of stretch of a muscle in which they are embedded (see Figure 2.8). If a muscle is being overstretched the spindle will cause the motor unit to fire and contract the muscle. This will prevent the muscle from being stretched further and injured. The slight tightness that is felt whenever a muscle is stretched is the motor nerve stimulating the muscle to contract against the stretch. It is for this reason that bouncy, ballistic or 'double flex' movements are not recommended, especially at end of range of motion.

Golgi Tendon Organs

These proprioceptors are located near the junction of the muscle and tendon fibres (see Figure 2.9). The Golgi tendon organs are activated mainly by the stretch placed upon them by the contraction of the muscles in whose tendons they lie. In other words, in contrast to the spindles, stimulation of the Golgi tendon organs results in the inhibition of the muscles in which they are located. This can be interpreted as a protective function in that during attempts to lift extremely heavy loads that could cause injury, the tendon organs effect a relaxation of the muscles.

It should be pointed out that the spindles and tendon organs work together, the former causing just the right degree of muscular tension to effect a smooth movement and the latter causing muscular relaxation when the load is potentially injurious to the muscles and related structures.

Joint Receptors

These receptors are found in tendons, ligaments, bone, muscle and joint capsules. They supply information concerning the joint angle, the acceleration of the joint and the degree of pressure placed on the joint.

All of the above proprioceptors plus other receptors (e.g. sight and sound) are used to give us a sense of awareness of body and limb position, as well as to provide us with automatic reflexes concerned with posture.

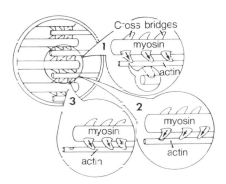

Fig. 2.7: Muscle Movement Sequence: (1) cross bridges extend towards actin; (2) cross bridges pull the actin forward; (3) stimulation ceases, connection is broken and cross bridges swivel back to next connection causing muscle to shorten

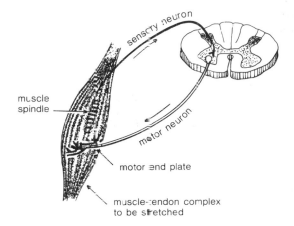

Fig. 2.8: The Muscle Spindle

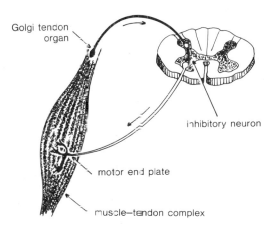

Fig. 2.9: The Golgi Tendon Organ

Muscle Fibre Types

Two distinct types of muscle fibre have been identified in human skeletal muscle. These are *fast twitch* (FT) and *slow twitch* (ST) fibres.

Fast twitch fibres are characterised by a quick response to stimulation. Physiologically, they have a high capability for anaerobic metabolism, especially in the production of ATP during the initial stages of glucose breakdown in glycolosis. Athletes in short term sprint-like activities use predominantly fast twitch fibres, but they are also important in the stop-and-go or change-of-pace sports like basketball or football which require rapid energy from anaerobic pathways.

Slow twitch fibres, on the other hand, have a slower contraction speed than fast twitch. As might be expected, they become activated in endurance activities, which depend almost entirely on the energy generated by aerobic metabolism. Long distance running is an example of an activity most suited to slow twitch fibre types. Middle distance running or swimming, or sports like basketball, hockey and soccer require a blend of both aerobic and anaerobic capacities, and they activate both types of muscle fibres in different proportions (see Table 2.3).

Table 2.3: Percentage of Fast and Slow Twitch Fibres in Various Activities

Activity	% Slow twitch	% Fast twitch	Predominant energy system
Sprint	30	70	phosphate
Middle Distance	60	40	lactate/aerobic
Marathon	80	20	aerobic
Weight Lifting	30	70	phosphate
Hockey	50	50	phosphate/lactate aerobic
Squash	60	40	aerobic/phosphate

Because of their differences in the use of oxygen, fast and slow twitch muscle fibres generally differ in colour. Slow twitch fibres are darker, usually red in colour, reflecting greater use of the oxygenated blood supply. Fast twitch fibres are usually white.

The differences are obvious in the different muscles of various animals. The legs of chicken, for example, are dark meat while the wings are white, reflecting the role of the legs in aerobic activity (walking) and the wings in brief spurts of anaerobic effort (flying).

Fast and Slow Twitch Fibres

As well as ST and FT, two other fibre types have been identified. Both are similar to FT fibres. Hence the main FT fibres are now called 'fast twitch a' (or IIa) and the others are called 'fast twitch IIb and IIc'.

FTc fibres have various amounts of ST and FT myosin and hence are thought to be a transitional form through which fibres may pass when transforming from type I to type II, and vice versa.

The four main types of fibre and their properties are shown in the following table.

Table 2.4: Properties of Muscle Fibre Types

Fibre type	Energy type	Contraction
Slow twitch I	Oxidative	Slow/fatigue resistant
Fast twitch IIc	Oxidative	Fast/fatigue resistant
Fat twitch IIa	Oxidative plus Glycolytic	Fast/intermediate fatiguability
Fast twitch IIb	Glycolytic	Fast/fatiguable

Research interest now centres around the effects of training on muscle fibre structure. Can a sprinter (with a high proportion of FT fibres), for example, increase ST fibres through endurance training? Or can an endurance athlete increase speed potential through intermediate high-intensive training?

Most research has looked at endurance training or stimulating muscle actions with electrical activity. Hence there's much to be done, still. But in general, findings indicate that:

• Both ST and FT fibres can increase their oxidative (aerobic) capacity through endurance training.
• Although not yet convincingly proven, it appears that some FT fibres (probably IIc) can take on ST characteristics. This suggests it may be possible to develop the endurance capacity of a 'sprinter' (i.e. someone with a high FT/ST ratio) through endurance training.
• Changes from ST to FT fibre are more difficult to achieve (if possible at all). This implies that 'sprint' ability can't be enhanced significantly.
• A sudden stop in training may reverse the changes in fibre type produced through training. The ratio of fibre typing appears to be largely genetically determined. However, it appears genetic endowment is of much more importance for sprint type events than for endurance activities.

Despite the classification outlined here, the distinction between fibre types is not clear cut. There is an overlap of most of the enzymes involved in both major types, and some classifications differentiate between up to 18 different fibre types.

Muscle Size

Gains in muscle size or *hypertrophy* usually accompany increases in strength or muscular endurance. The opposite, or *atrophy* of muscles, results from inactivity.

Until recently, increases in muscle size following weight training were thought to be due to an increase only in the size of fibres, rather than the number. However, recent research has shown that in some instances the number of fast twitch fibres is increased through a process known as 'longitudinal fibre splitting'.

Muscle hypertrophy following intensive weight training is thought to be a result of increased fibre number, increased fibre size, more total protein, and hypertrophy of connective, tendinous or ligamentous tissues.

Research also indicates that FT fibres respond more to strength training than do ST fibres, by increasing in size. This suggests that the individual suited to power and anaerobic activities (sprinting, throwing etc.) will tend to bulk more readily in response to resistance training than the individual suited to endurance. Because conversion of fibre types is unlikely (especially from ST to FT), this may imply that the endurance athlete will always have more difficulty adding muscle bulk.

Unlike the opposite, increases in muscle strength do not necessarily mean an increase in muscle size. This is especially so with women, because of the lack of the male hormone testosterone, which influences the development of muscle hypertrophy.

Muscle Soreness

Muscle soreness is usually attributed to the accumulation of lactic acid as a waste product in the muscles. This may only be true of acute soreness, where ischaemia, or a decrease in blood flow caused by intense exercise, doesn't allow for the quick removal of metabolic wastes such as lactic acid and potassium.

Delayed soreness usually occurs at least 12 hours after a person performs 'unfamiliar' or vigorous exercise. It can become more severe on the following day and then disappear after some 3–6 days. The causes aren't known, but a number of theories have been put forward. For example:

The pressure theory suggests that post-exercise wastes such as histamines build up in the muscles and cause pressure and thus pain. The theory is popular, particularly among weight lifters, but it has little scientific support.

The 'tear' theory proposes that pain is caused by micro-tears in muscle fibres following unaccustomed movement. Examination for chemicals in exercised muscles which could be indicative of tears, however, has shown that these exist independently of pain.

The spasm theory claims that the ischaemia caused by exercise results in the production of a pain substance (substance P) which stimulates nerve endings causing spasms which in turn cause further pain. The evidence in support of this remains contradictory.

The connective tissue theory is perhaps the most scientifically supported theory of muscle pain. This is based on observations that soreness is more common following negative (eccentric) muscle contractions than following positive (concentric) muscle contractions. Research indicates that negative contractions put a greater strain on a muscle's inelastic components (or connective tissue). This is supported by the observation that soreness is usually located in and around the tendon of an eccentrically contracted muscle.

The theory has also been supported by biopsies and electrical examinations of the tendons of eccentrically contracted muscles in animals and humans. However, the theory is thought by some researchers to be an insufficient explanation.

The Cardiorespiratory System and Training

The maintenance of life depends on the efficient operation of the body at the cellular level. Each cell needs a ready supply of oxygen and food, while carbon dioxide and other waste products must be carried away from it.

The heart and the lungs coordinate through the *pulmonary circulation system* where de-oxygenated blood is pumped from the right side of the heart (see Figure 2.10) via the pulmonary arteries to the lungs for oxygenation. (This is the only part of the circulatory system where de-oxygenated blood flows through arteries). Oxygenated blood is then returned to the left side of the heart via the pulmonary veins. (This is the only part of the circulatory system where oxygenated

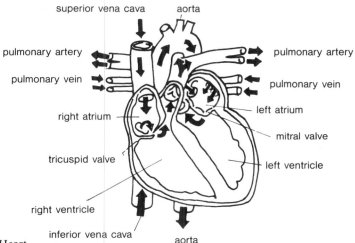

Fig. 2.10: The Human Heart

blood flows through veins.) Oxygenated blood is then pumped to the muscles and organs of the body through the *systemic circulation system*, whence de-oxygenated blood is returned to the right side of the heart.

Vigorous exercise increases the need of the muscle cells for oxygen and for removal of waste products. This means that the heart will have to beat faster, resulting in an increase in *cardiac output*, which increases the blood supply to the working muscle.

If sufficient oxygen does not get through to the muscles, and the intensity of the exercise is maintained, the additional energy requirements will come from the anaerobic system. This results in muscle fatigue through the accumulation of lactic acid. Long duration activity therefore, depends on the ability of the heart and lungs to deliver oxygen.

Cardiac Output

In order to fully meet the oxygen demands during exercise two major blood flow changes are necessary:

1. An increase in *cardiac output*, which is the amount of blood pumped by the heart each minute.
2. A redistribution of blood flow from inactive organs to the active muscles.

The increase in cardiac output during exercise is brought about through increases in (1) stroke volume, i.e., the amount of blood pumped by the heart each beat; and (2) heart rate, the number of times the heart beats per minute. Mathematically, the relationship of cardiac output ($\dot{Q}$) to stroke volume (S.V.) and heart rate (H.R.) is as follows:

$\dot{Q}$ (litres per minute) = S.V. (ml per beat) × H.R. (beats per min)

For example, if during heavy exercise stroke volume was 160 ml per beat and heart rate was 185 beats per minute, cardiac output would be:

$\dot{Q}$ = 0.16 litre per beat × 185 beats per min
  = 29.6 litres/min

As a result of an increase in cardiac output the heart will require fewer beats per minute, both during the exercise phase and at rest. This basic principle, an improvement in the capacity of the heart with training, is called a training effect.

Training Effect

The human body is a dynamic, responding organism capable of growth and development, atrophy and hypertrophy of tissues. As such, all systems and functions respond to both immediate (exercise) and chronic (training) demands placed upon them. By responding to the immediate elevated demands of exercise, the organs and systems stressed are forced to function at a level above that to which they are normally accustomed. This stimulus, when repeated at regular intervals of sufficient frequency, intensity and duration, produces a training effect enabling a higher than previous maximal training function.

Venous Return

Regardless of the mechanisms that increase cardiac output during exercise, the heart can pump only as much as it receives. For this reason, cardiac output is ultimately dependent on the amount of blood returned to the heart, in other words, upon the *venous return*.

The primary mechanism for increasing the venous return during exercise is the *muscle pump*. The muscle pump is the result of the mechanical pumping action produced by rhythmical muscular contractions. As the muscles contract, their veins are compressed and the blood within them is forced towards the heart. Blood is prevented from flowing backwards because the veins in the limbs contain numerous valves, which permit flow only towards the heart.

If the muscle pump is not working, as is the case when you stand still for a long time or immediately stop following a workout, then blood pooling occurs resulting in insufficient blood flow to the brain and fainting.

Heart Rates

While the average pulse rate of a sedentary man is around 72 bpm and of a woman around 80 bpm, these rates are often significantly less in trained athletes. Marathon runners have recorded resting heart rates as low as 35 bpm.

Heart rate responses to standard work loads have, over the years, been used as an indication of physical fitness capacities and changes. With training that raises the heart rate (HR) above a standard work load (often estimated from formulae using age and estimated maximal HRs), the working HR will decrease, enabling a greater work load to be carried out with the same effort. Heart rate, then, is an important feedback mechanism for any exerciser or exercise programmer as we shall see in Chapter 4.

Blood Vessels

During exertion there is a redistribution of blood flow from the organs of the body to the working muscles so that these receive a greater proportion of cardiac output. This redistribution of blood flow is dependent on the vasoconstriction (narrowing) of arterioles supplying the inactive parts of the body, such as the kidneys, liver and stomach, and the vasodilation (opening) of arterioles to the skeletal muscles being used in the activity. With training this whole system becomes more efficient, thereby always supplying skeletal muscles with sufficient blood flow.

Maximal pulse is the highest an individual's heart rate will go. This generally declines with age from around 220 bpm in under 20-year-olds to around 160 bpm in over 60-year-olds. Maximal pulse is also influenced by sex, with females generally having a slightly higher MPR than males.

Blood Pressure and Exercise

Systolic and diastolic pressure average around 120 mmHg and 80 mmHg respectively with a mean pressure of about 93 mmHg. The mean arterial pressure is the average of the systemic systolic and diastolic pressures during a complete cycle (systole plus diastole).

During exercise, blood pressure increases as a result of the accompanying increase in cardiac output. In fact, exercise affects systolic blood pressure more than diastolic or mean pressure. This is because during exercise there is a simultaneous decrease in resistance as a result of vasodilation of the arterioles supplying blood to the active skeletal muscles. This means that blood will drain from the arteries through the arterioles and into the muscle capillaries, thus minimising changes in diastolic pressure.

Maximal Oxygen Uptake

Maximal oxygen uptake (VO_2max), is the maximal amount of oxygen capable of being transported to and consumed by the working muscles. In other words, it can be used as a measure of fitness. At rest, the body uses about 3.5 millilitres of oxygen per kilogram of body weight per minute (3.5 ml/kg/min) to sustain life. The highest VO_2max recorded, that of a trained cross-country skier, was 92 ml/kg/min. A low VO_2max, indicating poor fitness in a middle aged man, would be around 26 ml/kg/min. Examples of VO_2max recordings are shown in Figure 2.11.

As physical fitness and the capacity of the heart improve with training, oxygen uptake will improve significantly. This can be demonstrated in tests of aerobic capacity.

Another measure of aerobic capacity is the Met, short for *Basic metabolic unit*. One Met is the amount of oxygen used by the body at rest (i.e. around 3.5 ml/kg/min), and maximal oxygen uptake is expressed in terms of multiples of this unit or max Mets. Met scores can be equated with VO_2max scores by multiplying Mets by 3.5. In training for cardiovascular improvement, exercises at a predetermined Met level (generally 60-80% of max Mets) are often used to ensure sufficient individual effort to establish a training effect.

Treadmill

Males

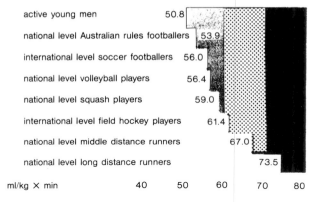

Females

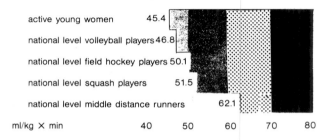

Fig. 2.11: Maximal Oxygen Uptake Values obtained on Australian sportsmen and sportswomen. (From Pyke and Roberts, University of W.A.)

A low intensity exercise class to music could have an exercise intensity of 8 Mets. Expressed as oxygen consumption this will be $8 \times 3.5 = 28$ ml/kg/min. Figure 2.12 outlines a Met scale of common activities. Using this measurement of energy expenditure (1 Met = 4.2 kJ or 1 Calorie), the maximum level attained by a sedentary middle-aged male is 10–12 Mets, increasing to 14–16 Mets for those who exercise regularly such as at high intensity classes and super-circuits.

Dehydration

Exercising in the heat can cause problems of excessive moisture loss. Dr David Costill for example has shown that marathon runners can lose in excess of 6 litres of sweat, even during an event conducted in cool conditions. The marathoner therefore has to be conscious of how to replace this fluid and what forms this replacement should take.

The dangers of heat disorders and dehydration are not just restricted to the endurance athlete, but to anyone exercising in hot or humid environments. It's feasible for an individual to lose 3–5 kilograms of water (1 kilogram equals 1 litre of water) during an advanced floor class or a circuit program lasting 1–1½ hours.

When the body loses excessive fluid, as can occur with dehydration, the blood becomes more viscous (thicker), and its ability to flow is significantly reduced. This results in an insufficient blood supply to the working muscles which consequently lose their ability to work aerobically. At this point either the effort must be reduced, or the muscles generate energy anaerobically, a process which can only be continued for a limited period of time.

Not replacing body fluids after exercise results in a feeling of lethargy and in some instances dizziness associated with an elevated heart rate. In some cases, fluid losses are even aimed at as a (misguided) means of losing weight. Water contains no calories however, hence the drinking of fluid will not affect body fat.

The body dissipates most of its heat through two primary avenues: vaso-dilation and evaporation.

Vaso-dilation refers to the arteries increasing in size (in contrast to decreasing in size, vaso-constriction) and taking warm blood from within the body to the periphery. The main disadvantage with this avenue of heat loss is that blood is directed away from the working muscle leading to oxygen debt.

Evaporation refers to the dissipation of heat from the body through the evaporation of sweat. In fact, the sweat that is seen dripping off the body does not cool the body. It is the sweat that is not seen (evaporated) that cools the body. For this reason exercising in a hot humid environment increases the risk of heat stress due to the amount of water vapour in the atmosphere (see Figure 2.13).

Finally, in regards to sweating, it should be noted that sweating is the most important avenue of heat loss. The old saying 'horses sweat, men perspire and women glow' is totally untrue as horses, men and women must sweat profusely if they wish to effectively control their body temperature.

Heat Stress and Anaerobic Threshold

Heat can effect performance in ways other than its straight effect on dehydration. Endurance performances are known to be influenced by both aerobic capacity and the anaerobic threshold (AnT).

AnT is that point at which muscle energy changes from being provided by predominantly aerobic sources

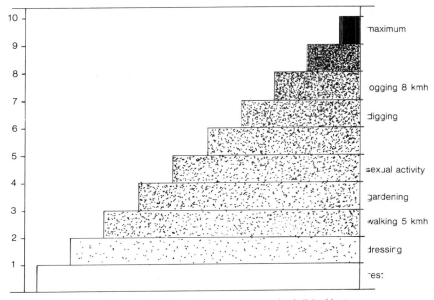

Using this measurement of energy (calorie) expenditure, the maximum level attained by a sedentary middle-aged male is 10–12 mets, increasing to 14–16 mets for those who exercise regularly such as by jogging or playing squash.

Fig. 2.12: Met Scale of Common Activities (from Heart Foundation, *Guide To Exercise*)

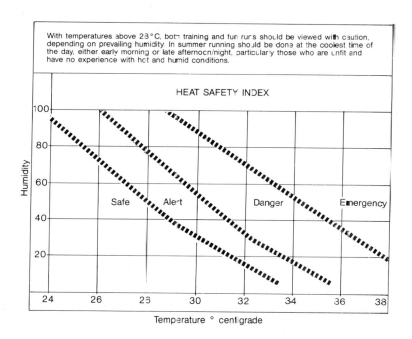

Fig. 2.13: Heat Stress Index (from Heart Foundation, *Guide to Exercise*)

(i.e. where oxygen is being continuously supplied and the individual doesn't get 'out of breath') to where it's provided predominantly by anaerobic sources (i.e. where breathing becomes heavy and exercise can't be continued indefinitely at that rate).

Although some research has been done on aerobic power in the heat, little has been carried out on the effects of heat on AnT.

Logically, some effect would seem obvious because more blood is diverted to the skin in the heat to allow for sweating and the cooling that results from evaporation. This would mean a decrease in blood flow (and hence oxygen) to the working muscles, which would then call on anaerobic (without oxygen) sources for energy.

Such was recently tested at the University of Western Australia. Using 9 trained cyclists together with 9 other active men with no significant cycling experience, Brian Dawson and Frank Pyke from UWA's Department of Human Movement Studies tested AnT by taking blood samples after the men had pedalled a bicycle at a set load in both hot (35 degrees C) and cool (21 degrees C) conditions in a special heat chamber.

AnT was reached more quickly in every case in the hotter conditions than in the cool. Also there was less of an effect for those trained cyclists than for the other, equally fit, but non-cyclist group.

In plain language this suggests that not only is it hard for an individual to last as long in an endurance event in the heat, it's also difficult to go as fast. Training may improve this, but the effect is still marked.

Replacement of Fluid Losses

The natural desire for drinking water is not always adequate to the task of replacing a sufficient amount of fluid. Thus, the exercising person should be aware that the replacement of fluid should be done over a period of time and not in one 'drinking bout'.

According to studies carried out on the composition of body sweat, the main substance lost during exercise is water. In fact, up to 14% of the body's fluids can be lost in cooling the body—through sweat and evaporation. Water makes up approximately 60% of the total body weight and reductions in this volume can interrupt normal body activities.

As commonly thought, electrolyte substances (sodium, calcium, potassium, chloride, magnesium) are also lost in sweat, but not in the concentration at which they are found in body fluid. For example a 14% loss in body water in a marathon runner may be accompanied by an 8% loss in sodium. Replacement drinks which are concentrated at the level of body fluid will restore a higher proportion of sodium to the blood than exists in the steady state.

This in turn can lead to complications. Because sodium (salt) absorbs moisture, fluid which may be used for cooling purposes is less available, adding to the risks of dehydration and heat exhaustion. Accordingly, researchers recommend a dilution of commercial electrolyte—replacement drinks beyond that usually proposed by the manufacturers.

Alternatively, plain water as a replacement fluid during and after an exercise session is considered to be more than adequate. If a glucose solution is added for energy, this should be in a limited amount, because excess concentrations may slow down the rate of gastric emptying (i.e. increase the time taken for fluid to be passed through the system).

Other recommendations for fluid replacement are:

1. Drink 2 glasses (300–500 ml) of fluid 15–20 minutes before heavy exercise and one glass (150–250 ml) at 15–20 minute intervals throughout the activity. Continue drinking after exercise.

2. If competing in endurance activities (e.g. a marathon), take regular drinks at drink stops from the start. Because it takes time for fluids to pass through the system, these should be ingested before thirst is felt.

3. The most important consideration is the replacement of water. Adding small quantities (e.g. 1 g/litre) of salt and sugar may be useful in prolonged exercise (over 1 hour).

4. Drink fluids that are cool (10–15 degrees C) in order to speed emptying time from the stomach.

3 Principles of Exercise Programming

Exercise is a major factor in the maintenance of health of an individual. Among its proven benefits are:

1. Increased physical work capacity (strength, endurance).
2. Increased cardiovascular and respiratory efficiency.
3. Decreased risk of coronary heart disease.
4. Changes in body metabolism (e.g. reduced level of obesity).
5. Delay of physiological ageing effects.
6. Psychological effects (e.g. stress reduction, increased self-confidence).

Exercise programmes can be designed to develop one or a number of aspects of physical fitness. For example, there's fitness for cardiovascular (heart/lung) efficiency, for strength, speed, flexibility, muscle endurance, power, agility and balance.

Each aspect of fitness involves varying contributions of the energy systems discussed in Chapter 2. Which type of fitness is important will depend on the needs of an individual. A shot-putter, for example, will need strength and power but little agility, while a marathon runner would need heart/lung fitness and muscle endurance but not necessarily strength, agility or balance.

Training for specific purposes is covered in more detail in sports training texts. Here we're interested primarily in the types of fitness that will most benefit the non-competing population. In particular these are:

1. cardiovascular fitness *(stamina)*,
2. flexibility *(suppleness)*, and
3. muscular strength *(strength)*.

They've been called **the 3 S's** of fitness. We'll look at each in the chapters that follow.

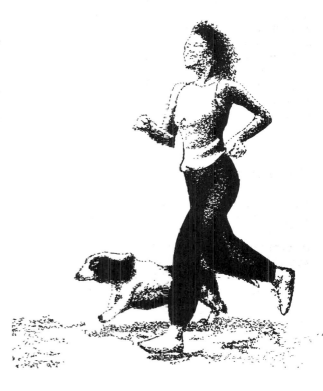

A minimum amount of exercise is required to produce a training effect

Principles of Exercise Prescription

The first step in exercise programming is to establish a specific objective; to determine which physical parameters are to be improved. If body weight and aerobic condition are important, aerobic exercise will be indicated. If muscle and joint stiffness is a problem, flexibility training should play a large part. If muscle strength is low, some strengthening work should be included.

Next, a program should be designed to meet the established objectives. This necessarily involves decisions about the *type, duration* and *frequency* of exercise as well as the means to evaluate progress in the form of relevant physiological and/or performance tests.

The Training Threshold

There is a minimum amount of exercise which is required to produce significant improvements in any physical fitness parameter. This is referred to as the *training threshold*. For example, the recognised training threshold for the development of aerobic fitness in most people is regarded as 20 minutes of effort at a heart rate of between 60% and 80% of maximum heart rate or MHR (see Chapter 4).

Aerobic/Anaerobic Thresholds

As well as the training threshold, there are thresholds for aerobic and anaerobic effort which are important for training purposes. Coaches for years have argued the benefits of fast, anaerobic work-outs in contrast to longer, slower aerobic training, particularly for middle-distance athletes.

Thresholds occur during the progression from low to maximum exercise. The first stage involves primarily aerobic metabolism and is characterised by heart rates below 130 beats per minute and only moderate increases in ventilation. Blood lactates (a sign of energy intensity) don't change much from resting values.

The second stage or *aerobic threshold* (AT), occurs at a point between 40-60% of a person's maximal oxygen uptake (VO_2 max). Heart rates rise to between 130-150 bpm and ventilation and blood lactate increase, but the effort can be kept up for 3-4 hours. At this level a person can carry on a conversation comfortably while exercising.

If the exercise is then increased, ventilation will increase sharply and heart rate and blood lactate will rise (see Figure 3.1). The effort can't be maintained for longer than a few minutes. This is the *anaerobic threshold* (AnT).

In endurance athletes AnT is all-important because performance above an established AnT will quickly lead to fatigue. Hence a marathon runner with a lower overall aerobic fitness may beat an aerobically fitter runner if he/she can maintain a higher AnT.

Overload

The *overload principle* also applies to training. This implies that an individual must exercise at a level above that which can be normally carried out comfortably. For example, to increase the strength of a muscle, it must be contracted against a greater than normal resistance. The intensity, duration and frequency of exercise, therefore, should be above the training threshold and be gradually but progressively increased as the body adapts to the increasing demands. As fitness levels improve, so the training threshold will be raised.

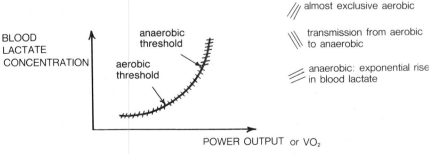

Fig. 3.1: The Relationship between Aerobic and Anaerobic Threshold

Specificity

The principle of *specificity* of training effect implies that different forms of exercise produce different results. The type of exercise carried out is specific both to the muscle groups being used and to the energy sources involved. For example, there is little *transfer of training* from strength training to the cardiovascular system. Similarly, prolonged running is unlikely to improve endurance swimming performances.

This was demonstrated in a series of experiments carried out by Dr Frank Katch and Dr William McArdle at Queens College in New York. A group of 20 men were trained on a bicycle ergometer over an 8-week period and tested before and after on both the bicycle ergometer and a treadmill. Maximal oxygen uptake improved 7.8% as measured by the bicycle, but only 2.6% as measured on the treadmill.

In another study, swimming was used as the primary training technique over 10 weeks and subjects were tested before and after on swimming and running (treadmill) tests. Results showed an improvement of 11% in VO_2 max. as measured by the swimming test, but no improvement in the treadmill. Improvements in this case were apparently so specific as to be non-transferable to exercise involving other large muscle groups.

Reversibility

Training effects are reversible in that if workouts stop and are not done often enough or with sufficient intensity, benefits can be lost quickly. This can be prevented by continuing training at a maintenance level after a high level of conditioning has been obtained.

Progression

As a person becomes more fit, a higher intensity of exercise is required to create an overload and therefore provide continued improvements. This is most pertinent for athletes who wish not merely to maintain a good level of fitness but to improve on that level. Progression can be through either increased intensity or duration of exercise sessions.

Warm-Up

Every exercise session should be preceded by a period of *warm-up* where the body is prepared gradually for the effort to come. Warm-up should be gentle and rhythmic and preferably use the muscles to be involved in the major activity. It should take up 10–20% of the time spent in the primary exercise.

Cool-Down

As with the warm-up, a *cool-down* period should be a vital component of an exercise session. This involves a gradual decrease in the intensity of the exercise until the body's physiological functions return to the resting state. An adequate cool-down helps the muscles of the body return blood to the heart rather than pool in the muscles.

Types of Exercise Programs

For the purposes of this book we'll be looking at training programs for the 3 S's—*stamina, suppleness* and *strength*. Only a general run-down of each will be given here. More detailed exercise programs will be covered in Chapters 4, 5 and 6.

Cardiorespiratory Training (Stamina)

Cardiorespiratory fitness is often called *aerobic* fitness because it involves predominantly aerobic energy. It is usually regarded as the most important aspect of community fitness because of its relationship to coronary heart disease (CHD) and weight control.

People who regularly exercise aerobically have a lower incidence of coronary heart disease than those who remain sedentary. In fact, according to Dr Ralph Paffenbarger, Professor of Epidemiology at Stanford University, who has carried out much research into the benefits of exercise: '...*strenuous and continual exercise provides the greatest protection (with the possible exception of lowered blood pressure) against death from heart disease.*'

Of course any exercise, if not carried out properly, can be dangerous *for some people*. In cases where heart disease is advanced for example, sudden excessive exertion may bring on heart failure. Yet the chances of these events occurring in a healthy person are minute. To understand just how much so, we need to look at some statistics.

The Dangers of Exercise

According to Dr Roy Shephard, Professor of Preventive Medicine at the University of Toronto in Canada, the chances of a normal man having a heart attack during one half hour session of heavy exercise is 1 in 5 million. In a normal woman, the chance is 1 in 17 million.

The most detailed Australian study of sudden deaths has shown that in only 7% of cases was death associated with strenuous exercise. The other 93% occurred while the victim was carrying out everyday activities such as standing, sitting still or lying down.

Similarly, Dr Ernst Jokl in his book on *Exercise and Cardiac Death* points out that sudden deaths do not occur in persons with a healthy heart. Says Jokl: 'Not one instance was encountered in which death could be regarded as due to the effects of extreme exertion on a previously healthy heart.'

Exercise does have risks, particularly for the previously sedentary person. But these need to be weighed against the risks of *not* exercising. Then a decision can be made as to which is the more dangerous path to take.

Developing Aerobic Fitness

To develop 'aerobic' fitness, it is necessary to exercise at an intensity above the training threshold (generally around 60% of the maximum heart rate) for a period of 15–60 minutes, on 3–5 days each week. Exercise may be continuous such as with LSD (long slow distance) training, or it may be intermittent where intervals of exercise are interspersed with periods of rest or mild exercise *(interval training). Circuit training* is another form of aerobic conditioning which also includes aspects of strength and flexibility.

In circuit training, the individual is given a variety of exercises to do continuously. While the exercises in isolation may not be aerobic, in continuous movement they readily become so. Examples of established circuit training routines are the 5BX and XBX plans and many of the modern aerobic dance routines.

Continuous exercise may be more appropriate for individuals with low fitness levels, while intermittent exercise is seen as being superior for preparing an athlete for competitive sports where aerobic fitness is important.

Aerobic Conditioning Guidelines

Some basic rules for the development of aerobic fitness are:

1. If you don't exercise regularly, are over 35 years of age or have any major health problems (see Chapter 4), have a medical examination before starting an exercise program.

2. Warm up gradually at the start of each session and cool down gradually at the end. Stretching exercises (see Chapter 5) should immediately follow the general warm-up session.

3. Carry out physical activity involving large muscle groups, e.g. jogging, swimming, cycling, etc.

4. Start the program slowly and increase the intensity, duration and frequency of exercises gradually until they conform to prescription.

5. Avoid sudden exercise of unaccustomed intensity. Any change of activity should be gradual.

6. Wear good-fitting, appropriate shoes if running.

7. Use your heart rate as a guide to the intensity of exercise.

More details of aerobic conditioning are covered in Chapter 4.

Flexibility Training (Suppleness)

Flexibility training involves stretching of muscles and tendons to maintain or increase suppleness.

Stretching can be of three major types:

1. *Static stretching:* which involves the gradual lengthening of a muscle to a stretched position where it is held.

2. *PNF stretching:* PNF (proprioceptive neuromuscular facilitation) stretching is a form of static stretching incorporating isometric contraction of the stretched muscle. In essence, this means applying an immovable force to a stretched muscle which may, in turn, help to lengthen than muscle. PNF stretching is the type

now recommended by most sports medicine experts for flexibility and injury prevention.

3. *Ballistic stretching:* Often called 'dynamic' stretching, this involves bouncing or movement at the point of maximum expansion. It is not recommended because it can result in injury due to the stretch reflex (see Chapter 2). If over-stretching through bouncing occurs, the result may be a tightening of the muscle rather than the desired loosening.

A high degree of flexibility is desirable for some activities and a reasonable degree is important for the prevention of soft tissue injuries. An adequate warm-up which involves large muscle groups and whole body movements should precede stretching.

Flexibility is highly joint specific, meaning that a high degree of flexibility in one joint doesn't necessarily mean that the same degree of flexibility will exist in other joints. To improve flexibility, the muscle should be stretched beyond its normal length.

More details on flexibility training are given in Chapter 5.

Muscle Training (Strength)

As we saw in Chapter 2, there are two main types of muscle fibre: fast twitch and slow twitch. Fast twitch fibres are used predominantly in strength and power activities, while slow twitch fibres are used in aerobic exercise. Strength training which involves high resistances usually develops the fast twitch fibres selectively.

Muscular endurance training can also be carried out with weights or resistance. The appropriate regimen is low-resistance exercise repeated many times.

Strength and endurance training may be *isotonic, isometric,* or *isokinetic.* All three methods have been shown to be effective, but since strength development is highly specific, the nature of the performance to be improved should determine the method adopted.

Isotonic training involves the contraction of a muscle against a moveable resistance (e.g. conventional or free weights). Contraction may occur while the muscle is shortening, in which case it is called a *concentric* (or positive) contraction (e.g. the biceps while raising a weight), or while the muscle is lengthening, in which case it is called an *eccentric* (or negative) contraction (e.g. the biceps while lowering a weight).

Isometric training involves static muscle contractions against an immovable resistance, e.g. pushing against a solid wall.

Isokinetic training involves contractions against a maximum resistance throughout the full range of movement. This is based on the principle that a muscle exerts different force at different stages in a contraction. In theory, to work the muscle maximally throughout the contraction requires a continuous monitoring of muscle movement and a variable adjustment of resistance at each stage of the movement.

Certain computerised rehabilitation equipment such as **Cybex** works on the isokinetic principle. Other systems such as **Nautilus** which is based on a cam system, and **Hydra-Fitness**, which is hydraulic, are often reported to be isokinetic. However, because they take little account of individual differences in muscle length etc., they are not truly isokinetic. Terms such as **Powernetic** have been used by some manufacturers to describe the different systems.

Exercise Equipment

For strength development, intensity is the important variable, whereas for muscular endurance the duration of exercise assumes more importance.

In both strength training and aerobic conditioning it's often useful to use effort against resistance. This can range from resistance of the body against its own weight to complicated isokinetic machinery.

Some of this equipment is good; some not so good. In rating the equipment shown in Table 3.1, the following criteria were used to arrive at a summary of their usefulness:

1. Effectiveness, i.e. for improving aerobic fitness; strength, power sport skills or muscle bulk; flexibility and body tension; lowering body fat content.

2. Safety.
3. Ability to maintain motivation.
4. Practicality and mechanical soundness.

Non-Exercise Machines: These include such things as vibrating belts, vibrating pads, rollers, electric stimulators and sauna suits.

Because no effort is required by the exerciser, the only effect these machines have is (perhaps) relaxation. Research has shown for example that a person using a vibrating belt for 15 minutes every day for a year can expect to lose about 0.5 kg of body fat in that year— little more than would be lost standing still for the same amount of time.

According to the American Medical Association: *'The so called effortless exercisers have a value limited to the intensity and duration of the movement they demand. They do not provide any hidden benefits or values. Their most serious shortcoming is that most of them do very little to improve the fitness of the heart and lungs which are most in need of exercise today.'*

Weight training equipment: There are now many different forms of weight training equipment ranging from the traditional barbell/dumbells to elaborate systems like **Hydra-fitness, Nautilus** and **Universal.**

The latter all operate on slightly different bio-mechanical principles. All have their advantages and disadvantages and all can be excellent forms of conditioning if used properly.

Impartial research shows that all systems are successful in the development of strength. The extent of improvement, however, depends on the measure of strength being used. If strength is assessed by variable resistance techniques, variable resistance training leads to approximately 20% greater improvement than constant resistance.

Table 3.1: Rating the Fitness Equipment

Item	Claimed Benefits	Advantages	Disadvantages	Rating (out of 10)
Exercise bikes	Fitness/weight loss	Convenient, functional, useful for obese and arthritics	Can get boring, often poorly built	9
Treadmills	Fitness/weight loss	Indoor use in cold climates, functional, maximal exercise	Expense, can get boring, can cause joint soreness	8½
Rowing machines	Fitness/weight loss/strength	Good all round exercise, uses upper body, not space consuming	Resistance can't be altered, can be boring, expense	8
Weights	Strength/power/body bulk/fitness	Versatility, able to vary programs, wide range of equipment, fitness and strength component	Dangers if used incorrectly, space, expense	8½
Mini-trampolines	Fitness	Novelty, less stress on weak joints of the lower limbs, not overly exerting for the less fit	Possible injury, motivation over a prolonged period	5½
Skipping rope	Fitness/weight loss	Low cost, convenient	Boring, possible joint injuries	7
Saunas, Steam baths, Swirl pools	Weight loss/tension release	Relaxing	Do not lose weight, dangerous for some, i.e. with heart deficiencies, high blood pressure, may cause infections, allergies	1
Passive exercise equipment (rollers, pads, electric caps, sauna suits, etc.)	Weight loss	Minor massage effect	Some dangers, e.g. in pregnancy; no effect on weight or fitness, almost totally useless	½

If assessment is through constant resistance techniques, the opposite is true. Improvements in body dimensions have also been shown to be roughly similar using fixed or variable resistance techniques. Hence the advantages claimed by various manufacturers do not always stand up to scrutiny.

Weights can be used for developing strength (heavy weights with low repetitions), building body bulk (heavy to medium weights with 6–10 repetitions), or developing cardiovascular fitness (light weights with high repetitions).

Traditionally, resistance equipment has been avoided by women because of the fear of developing muscle bulk. It is now accepted that large muscle development in women is limited by the lack of the male hormone testosterone and awareness of this is now leading to a greater involvement of women in body-shaping weight training programs.

Exercise bikes: In the gymnasium setting these are of the stationary type, but similar principles apply to moving bicycles.

Bikes can contribute an aerobic component to an exercise program. They can also be used for warming up and cooling down and for this reason alone are useful in an exercise area in a confined space.

Bikes can improve general fitness and strength in the thighs, knees and hips. They can reduce body fat and are especially useful for the obese or arthritic because they help support body weight.

Treadmills: An alternative to stationary cycling is stationary jogging. Treadmill running offers the advantages of ordinary running. It's a good form of cardiovascular conditioning and can help burn up body fat if carried out long enough.

As with exercise bicycles, the main disadvantage of treadmills is the problem of maintaining motivation. They are useful for warm-up and cool-down exercises in an indoor setting, but hold no other advantages over outdoor jogging.

Rowing machines: Rowing is an excellent form of aerobic exercise. It has the added advantage over running and cycling in that it uses the upper body and therefore increases the work effort and can contribute to upper body strength.

The problem of motivation noted above, however, is also true for rowing machines. For anyone but an experienced rower, the exercise can become boring over time—and this is not conducive to continued use.

Mini-trampolines: Mini-trampolines (sometimes called rebounders) are becoming popular in home exercise programs as well as in gymnasia because of the introduction of reasonably cheap home varieties.

Research has shown that some aerobic benefit can come from extended bouncing, although this is probably less than many manufacturers would claim. Work by Dr Victor Katch for example, indicates that the intensity of rebounding is about equivalent to running at 13–15 minute mile pace.

Similarly, Dr Larry Gettman says that the energy cost of rebounding is between 50–60% of that required to run on a treadmill at the same rate. Professor Bud Getchell, author of *Physical Fitness: A Way of Life*, claims that rebounding is . . .a nice way for sedentary people to start exercising, but not intense enough for someone who has reached a reasonable level of fitness'.

Clearly, the benefits gained are determined by the effort put in. But for older people and/or those who don't like exercising out of doors, mini-trampolines are functional—even if they're not the miracle machines some manufacturers claim.

Skipping ropes: Skipping is an exercise that's often regarded as the epitome of fitness. However, despite its long-term popularity, there have only been a limited number of scientific studies on its usefulness.

Those that have been done question its overall effect. Dr Bud Getchell, for example, has pointed out that more energy is expended at a given exercise heart rate in jogging than skipping (at a heart rate of 70–80 bpm). This is because the energy requirement of an activity is largely dependent on the amount of muscle involved in that activity. Jogging apparently uses more muscles than skipping in place, which accounts for the higher energy expenditure while jogging.

In a more recent series of studies from Kent State University, blood lactate measures as well as oxygen uptake have been taken to test the involvement of different energy systems in skipping. The findings indicate that while five minutes of skipping at a rate of between 120–160 bpm can be quite strenuous, much of the energy used comes from anaerobic rather than aerobic sources. The resultant build-up of lactic acid in the blood stream means that the exercise can't be continued for long at that rate.

The implications are that it may be difficult to skip at a level which would give an effect equivalent to jogging for a period long enough to provide a training effect. In the gym situation it may be useful for warming up or as part of a circuit routine. It's unlikely, however, that it can be kept up long enough to be useful alone as a conditioning technique.

4 Exercise Programming for Aerobic Conditioning

Although training and conditioning programs must be tailored to the individual, some basic principles apply for all people. In the first place, as we saw in Chapter 3, the most relevant type of exercises for the majority of the population are those defined by the 3S's: stamina, suppleness and strength. In this chapter we'll concentrate on principles of stamina development, or aerobic conditioning. In Chapters 5 and 6 we'll look at suppleness and strength development.

Prescribing Aerobic Programs

In recent years, there's been a vast amount of research aimed at clarifying issues concerning physical activity. Basically, this can be summarised under the four headings with the acronym FITT (Frequency, Intensity, Time and Type).

Frequency

In order to improve cardiovascular efficiency, a regular program of aerobic exercise should be carried out. Irregular mild exercise such as golf or doubles tennis is ineffective in developing high levels of aerobic fitness.

Research has shown that above average fitness can be maintained with regular workouts 3–4 times per week. Obviously more regular exercise will mean a higher level of fitness. However, for beginning exercisers, this will have a training effect without causing significant discomfort or boredom.

During endurance training, total body mass and fat weight (FW) are reduced, while lean body mass (LBM) generally remains constant or increases slightly. Programs designed for fat loss should be carried out

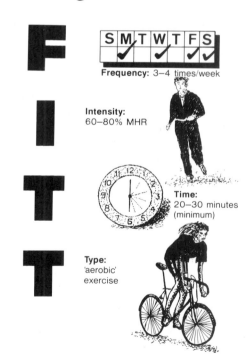

Frequency: 3–4 times/week

Intensity: 60–80% MHR

Time: 20–30 minutes (minimum)

Type: 'aerobic' exercise

Fig. 4.1: Principles of Exercise Programming

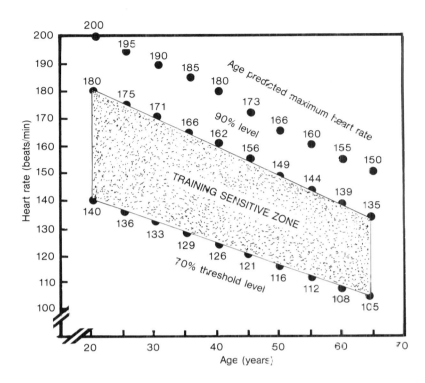

Fig. 4.2: Maximal Heart Rate Target Zone for use in aerobic exercise training (From Pyke, 1980)

on a minimum of three days a week, for twenty minutes a time at an intensity designed to expend approximately 1320 kJ (300 calories). A similar effect can be gained with an energy expenditure of 880 kJ (200 calories) per session if the exercise frequency is at least 4 days per week.

In order to maintain a training effect, exercise must be continued on a regular basis. There will be a significant reduction in fitness after two weeks of inactivity, with participants losing approximately 50% of their fitness after 4–12 weeks and 100% after 10–30 weeks.

Intensity

Because heart rate increases linearly with exercise effort, this is often used as a measure of the required intensity of exercise. Work carried out in Finland in the late 1950s showed that for noticeable gains in fitness, the heart rate during exercise should be raised by approximately 60% of the difference between the resting and maximal heart rates. Other formulae set the training range at between 70–85% of the estimated HR maximum. For individuals of various ages this is determined as shown in Figure 4.2.

Heart Rate and Exercise Intensity

Heart rate can be monitored easily by periodically taking the pulse during an exercise session and then adjusting the exercise intensity to bring the heart rate to a recommended level. This recommended heart rate level is called the *target heart rate*. In most community based exercise programs the two most common methods of determining desired exercise intensity are the Karvonen formula and the PRE Scale (perceived rate of exertion).

The Karvonen Formula

The Karvonen Formula is a relatively accurate method of determining target heart rate. The formula calculates a percentage of the *heart-rate reserve*, which is the difference between the resting heart rate and maximal heart rate.

The steps for the Karvonen Formula are as follows:

1. Determine RHR = _____ BPM

2. $\dfrac{}{\text{Max HR}} - \dfrac{}{\text{RHR}} = \dfrac{}{\text{HR Res}}$

3a. $\dfrac{\rule{2cm}{0.4pt}}{\text{HR Res}} \times \dfrac{0.60}{\text{Low level}} = \rule{2cm}{0.4pt} + \dfrac{\rule{2cm}{0.4pt}}{\text{RHR}} = \dfrac{\rule{2cm}{0.4pt}}{\text{THR}}$

3b. $\dfrac{\rule{2cm}{0.4pt}}{\text{HR Res}} \times \dfrac{0.70}{\text{High level}} = \rule{2cm}{0.4pt} + \dfrac{\rule{2cm}{0.4pt}}{\text{RHR}} = \dfrac{\rule{2cm}{0.4pt}}{\text{THR}}$

4a. $\dfrac{\rule{2cm}{0.4pt}}{\text{THR Low}} \div 6 = \dfrac{\rule{2cm}{0.4pt}}{\text{THR for 10 seconds}}$

4b. $\dfrac{\rule{2cm}{0.4pt}}{\text{THR High}} \div 6 = \dfrac{\rule{2cm}{0.4pt}}{\text{THR for 10 seconds}}$

Abbreviations:

BPM	=	Beats per minute
RHR	=	Resting heart rate
MAX HR	=	Maximum heart rate
HR Res	=	Heart rate reserve
THR	=	Training heart rate
Where		Maximal heart rate = 220 − age

Maximal heart rate is the highest heart rate a person can attain during heavy exercise. The most accurate way of determining maximal heart rate is to undergo a graded exercise test. In most instances this is not practical so the age predicted maximum heart rate formula of 220 − age is commonly used.

Using the Karvonen Formula calculate a lower 60% heart rate range and an upper 70% heart rate range for a 42 year old person with a resting heart rate of 85 bpm. At 60% intensity your answer should be 141 bpm or 23 bpm for a 10 second count and at 70% intensity your answer should be 150 bpm or 25 bpm for a 10 second count.

The Karvonen formula is an accurate way of determining target heart rate, with an error of ±5 to 10 beats per minute, and is recommended by the American College of Sports Medicine.

Perceived Rate of Exertion (PRE Scale)

Intensity of effort can also be determined by *Perceived Rate of Exertion Scales* (see Figure 4.3) developed by Gunner Borg. These scales are especially relevant to those people who may have an unusually low or high heart rate or those people that are on some form of medication that affects working heart rate. The PRE scales provide a means of quantifying subjective exercise intensity and have been found to correlate well (0.08 to 0.09) with oxygen uptake and heart rate.

The PRE chart should be placed in easy view of the exercising person, who should then be queried regularly as to the level of perceived exertion. Unless something out of the ordinary comes up, exercise is considered to be maximal or near maximal when the exerciser reports a perceived exertion of 9 to 10.

0	Nothing at all	5	Strong
0.5	Very, very weak	7	Very strong
1	Very weak	8	
2	Weak	9	
3	Moderate	10	Very, very strong
4	Somewhat strong		Maximal

The Talk Test

Another simple test of intensity is to ensure that the heart rate reaches a count of 120–130 bpm during exercise. This sets a safe lower value for the establishment of a training effect at most ages. At the higher level, the 'talk test' can be used to assess whether an individual is working out too hard. If the exerciser can't comfortably talk (or whistle) while exercising, the effort is more than likely anaerobic and therefore of greater intensity than necessary for safe training. For beginning exercisers it is unwise to continue at this level.

Pulse Taking Techniques

The most common errors that occur in recording intensity using heart rate include miscounting and taking too long to begin counting. Therefore, fitness instructors should be familiar with all the procedures for taking heart rates.

The two most common places for recording heart rate are the wrist and the neck.

1. Wrist The radial pulse can be felt on the radial artery of the wrist, in line with the thumb. Place the tips of the index and middle fingers (not the thumb, which has a pulse of its own) and press down slightly.

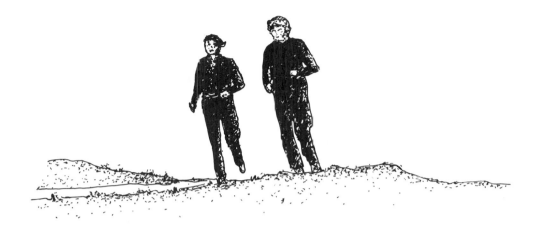

2. Neck The carotid pulse can be felt on the carotid artery, which is located on the neck just to the side of the throat. Place the first two fingers gently on the side of the neck. Too much pressure placed on the carotid artery may stimulate a reflex mechanism that causes the heart to slow down.

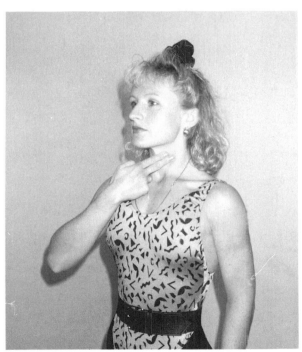

The pulse can be taken for 6 seconds (and multiplied by 10), for 10 seconds (and multiplied by 6), or for 15 seconds (and multiplied by 4).

It is recommended that the first pulse be counted as 1 and the pulse be taken for 10 seconds. If all instructors use this procedure then there will be consistency in the industry. Because heart rate begins to decrease soon after exercise stops, instructors should begin the count as soon as possible, preferably within 5 seconds.

Time

The minimum length of time of an exercise session for aerobic benefit is 15-20 minutes. Improved performance will continue (within reason) the longer the exercise session is continued. Beyond an hour, the returns start to become less. It is at this level that one might train if competition is the desired end.

For a beginning exerciser, it's often unwise to continue an exercise session beyond 30 minutes at the intensity prescribed above. Sessions should be limited to 15-20 minutes. If necessary, recovery periods of 1-2 minutes can be included between the heavier segments of activity.

Type

The type of aerobic activities that develop cardiovascular endurance are those that can be carried out continuously at a sustained rate (e.g. aerobically). The relative values of various activities depend on the amount of effort required (see Table 4.1). For example, golf, bowls, archery and doubles tennis may be recreational and enjoyable, but they do little for aerobic fitness. Vigorous, continuous and rhythmic activities on the other hand, like swimming, jogging, cross country skiing, cycling, canoeing, dancing and brisk walking are all potentially aerobic if carried out to the FITT formula.

A wide variety of aerobic activities can be carried out either individually or in groups. For example:

Table 4.1: Rating (out of 10) for a variety of exercise effects

	Weight control	Sleep	Digestion	Cardio-vascular endurance	Approx. energy use per minute (calories)[1]
Walking	6	6	5	6	5–7
Jogging	10*	8*	6	10*	12–16
Swimming	8	8*	7*	10*	6–11
Cycling	9	8*	6	10*	8–15
Tennis	6	5	6	7	5–11
Golf (walking)	3	3	5	4	5–8
Skiing (downhill)	8	8*	6	8	6–10
Stepping/Skipping/Jumping	7	5	5	7	5–11
Surfing	8	8*	7*	10*	6–11
Dancing	7	7	7*	7	4–11
Calisthenics	6	6	5	5	4–10
Handball/Squash	9	6	7*	10*	10–15
Canoeing	7	8*	6	8	4–10

* Signifies the best exercise(s) for that purpose.
[1] Energy use increases with body weight. These figures are based around an approximate body weight of 70 kg.

On Your Own

These are the simplest forms of activity because they don't require dependence on another person. They generally call for little elaborate equipment or expense, and can help an individual feel in control of his/her own programming.

Activities include: **walking, jogging, cycling, swimming, skating, weight training, skipping, trampolining, golf, rowing.**

Comparisons of some of these (e.g. running and swimming) as training techniques have shown that where equivalent intensities are used (i.e. equal exercise heart rates), both are equally efficient in developing cardiovascular fitness, although it has been estimated that the distance ratio between running and swimming is roughly 5:1; that is, 5 miles run equals 1 mile swum.

Follow the Leader

Many aerobic activities provide the stimulation of a group working out under the direction of an inspired leader. These may be indoor or outdoor, and with or without the added benefit of music. Classes are most suitable for those who prefer social interaction, who find it tedious organising their own routines, and who respond best to the motivating influences of others.

Activities include: **calisthenics, floor classes, dancercise, aquarobics, modern dance, ballet, synchronised swimming, karate.**

Studies of disco dancing carried out in Canada have shown that the effort required over ninety minutes of dancing is equivalent to an extended bout of jogging or cycling. Where heart rates are elevated to 120–140 bpm, the energy required is roughly equivalent to running at around 10 minute mile pace. This type of dancing is twice as strenuous as more traditional dancing, but perhaps less so than aerobic exercise to music.

One on One

For some people, competition provides the motivation for aerobic activity. Competitive games are also often a source of fun and enjoyment which can help to develop reflexes and specific skills as well as general aerobic fitness. The key to adequate aerobic exercise through competitive games is for both competitors to be similar in standard. This ensures that players are then kept continuously active.

Activities include: **tennis, squash, badminton, racquetball, handball, table tennis, wrestling, athletics, boxing.**

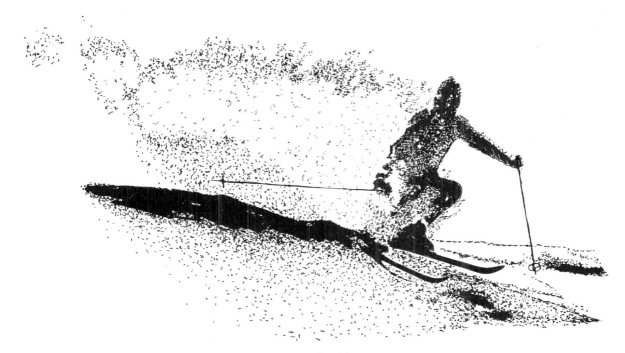

For a person to continue to exercise, that exercise must be enjoyable

Evaluation of the energy components of various racquet sports shows that these are of varying value in improving aerobic fitness. Singles tennis, for example, may be a reasonable way for a beginner to improve initial fitness levels, but will not sufficiently overload someone of advanced fitness. Squash, handball and badminton, conversely, are beneficial for skilled players who can keep the ball in play, but less so for beginners.

Team Games

Team sports combine the benefits of class activities and competitive games. Like class activities, they turn fitness into a social event, and the competitive element can be extremely stimulating.

Activities include: **basketball, volleyball, soccer, football, touch football, hockey, cricket, netball, water polo, softball, surf-lifesaving.**

In many of these (e.g. volleyball, cricket, softball), the action is stop-go; hence significant anaerobic or phosphate components are involved. Thus these games, while providing social stimulation, are not good fitness builders. Best for aerobic conditioning are those games that require constant movement throughout the game, e.g. soccer, hockey, basketball, water polo.

Getting Away

Certain outdoor activities combine adventure, fresh air and open skies with fitness-enhancing activity. These can vary according to season, location and availability of time. However, to be effective aerobic conditioners they should be carried out regularly (i.e. a minimum of three times a week), or combined with other events.

Activities include: **skiing, surfing, mountain climbing, bush-walking, orienteering, canoeing, rowing, and wind-surfing.**

Research has shown that cross-country skiing (langlaufing) is perhaps the best form of aerobic conditioning available. It rates even higher than jogging because of the use of the large muscles of the arms as well as of the legs. Downhill skiing rates less highly because of its stop-start nature and the short intense periods involved.

For an individual to continue an exercise program over a lifetime, that program has to be enjoyable. Hence, selection of the appropriate exercise is important. This can be done from a detailed interview or through completion of a questionnaire such as that shown in Figure 4.4.

Instructions:

1. Circle the number under each exercise corresponding to the answer in each category. Add scores down the column for each exercise to get your TOTAL TEST SCORES.

PERSONAL DETAILS	Jogging	Cycling	Swimming	Dancing	Skipping	Ball games
Age:						
Under 35	0	0	0	0	0	0
35–49	0	0	0	1	3	4
50–59	2	3	0	3	5	5
60+	4	7	0	4	8	6
Body Frame:						
Small/medium	0	0	0	0	0	0
Large	3	0	0	2	4	2
ARE YOU						
...more than a little overweight?						
No	0	0	0	0	0	0
Yes	4	3	0	4	5	6
...an indoor or outdoor type person?						
Indoor	7	6	4	0	0	4
Outdoor	0	1	2	0	5	0
...self-conscious about exercising in public?						
No	0	0	0	0	0	0
Yes	5	4	4	7	0	5
...competitive?						
very	3	5	3	8	8	0
moderately	0	4	3	5	5	2
not very	0	2	3	0	0	8
...prepared to pay more than $10 a week to exercise?						
Yes	0	0	0	0	0	0
No	0	2	1	4	0	4
...suffering limiting injuries to any of the following?						
Legs/ankles/knees	9	4	1	7	9	7
shoulders/arms	1	2	3	2	4	5
hip	9	3	3	7	8	7
back	5	5	2	6	5	6
...NOT within easy access (say 15 mins) of any of the following?						
pool/lake/sea	0	0	10	0	0	0
park/open space	5	0	0	0	0	0
gymnasium	0	0	0	3	0	4
sports facilities	0	0	0	0	0	10
safe bike routes	0	10	0	0	0	0
...prepared to give up daily time 3–4 days a week?						
less than 20 mins	4	5	10	10	3	10
20–40 mins	0	1	4	2	0	4
more than 40 mins	0	0	0	0	0	0
...a person who prefers....?						
exercising alone	0	0	0	5	0	10
exercising with a friend	1	2	2	0	3	0
exercising in group	2	4	2	0	6	0
TOTAL TEST SCORES						

2. Calculate your INTEREST SCORE for each activity.

If you think you'd enjoy carrying out the activity regularly, give yourself an INTEREST SCORE of 100.
If you think you may enjoy carrying out the activity regularly, give yourself an INTEREST SCORE of 90.
If the activity doesn't appeal give yourself an INTEREST SCORE of 80.

INTEREST SCORE

3. Calculate a FINAL SCORE for each activity by subtracting the TOTAL TEST SCORE from the INTEREST SCORE for each activity.

FINAL SCORE

4. The activity with the highest FINAL SCORE will generally be the most appropriate aerobic exercise for you. If there are several activities at the top falling within about 5 points of each other, choose the one you think you would prefer. Or combine them as part of the one program.

Fig. 4.4: Exercise Selector Questionnaire: Selecting the form of exercise most appropriate for an individual

Variety can also be important for motivation. A combination of aerobic activities carried out to the FITT plan will be as effective in developing cardiovascular conditioning as the continuation of one type of exercise only. For example, a typical fortnightly routine may be as follows:

	Week 1	Week 2
Monday	Jogging	Jogging
Tuesday	Swimming	Circuit training
Wednesday	Circuit training	Swimming
Thursday	Jogging	Jogging
Friday	Swimming	Circuit training
Saturday	Circuit training	Swimming
Sunday	–	–

In winter, an activity like cycling could substitute for swimming.

An added advantage to this type of program for a beginning exerciser is that it provides the opportunity for the exerciser, later, to select and concentrate on the most preferred type of exercise.

Exercise Prescription

Any exercise program must be fitted and evaluated on an individual basis. Anyone designing such a program should include the following considerations:

Age: The period of maximum maturity is between 25 and 30 with an acceleration in decline after age 50. As a person ages, improvement and recovery are slower, as are de-conditioning and re-conditioning. Prescription of exercise for the aged therefore must take into consideration the previous level of activity of the individual as well as any specific musculo-skeletal problems which may limit the type of exercises possible.

Sex: There are strength differences between men and women, but little apparent difference in muscular endurance. It has also been suggested that women only have between 80–90% of the aerobic capacity of men. When body weight and body fat are taken into consideration this difference seems to diminish.

Generally speaking, women are more flexible than men. Hence some stretching-type exercises used in modern floor classes, while suitable for the females in a class, can put extra strain on males. The competitive nature of many men also makes for added danger if the man doesn't accept his limitations.

Because of the absence of the male hormone testosterone, most women won't develop muscle bulking (hypertrophy) in response to exercise. In terms of cardiovascular function, women have a higher heart rate (5–10 bpm faster) than men.

Health Status: This will obviously determine the amount and intensity of overload and the rate of progression of an exercise program. Overload and intensity should be reduced even during minor illnesses such as a cold or minor infection. Since the body under such conditions is already under stress, further physical stress should be avoided.

Present Level of Condition: This will determine the starting point of an exercise program, and be reflected in the rate of improvement. The less fit a person is, the greater the improvement that can be shown. Conversely, the closer a person is to his or her maximum performance, the less improvement will be shown, and more effort will be required to make noticeable gains.

Previous Activity and Conditioning Experience: Although there are no residual benefits to exercise once a program has been discontinued, the individual who has had previous training experience is likely to respond more quickly to training than one who has not. That person will also usually achieve a higher level of fitness or skill.

Psychological Factors and Motivation: Each individual enters a training program with pre-determined perceptions regarding exercise, his or her level of skill, ability to learn and ability to endure a particular training regimen. Often the amount of improvement is limited more by psychological factors than by actual physical capacity. An instructor therefore must recognise and address this through motivational and human relations skills. Conversely, an individual's drive may exceed his or her physical capacities, and thus may have to be curbed.

Fitness Assessment: Objective fitness assessment is a key ingredient in any successful exercise program. A series of assessment tests that can be used in the practical situation is outlined in Chapter 10.

Individual Needs: Fitness evaluation procedures will establish specifically the areas of emphasis that need to be addressed in designing an exercise program. These include such things as time available, specific interests and health problems. These factors should all be assessed before prescribing an exercise program. The screening questionnaire shown in Figure 4.5 is one way of doing this as a supplement to the more detailed assessment tests of Chapter 10.

Pre-Activity Questionnaire

PERSONAL INFORMATION: Name _____

Age _____ Birth Date _____/ /_____ Sex M/F . . . .

Address _____

Phone _____ (Home) _____ (Bus)

Occupation _____ Employer _____

Emergency Contact: Name _____ Phone _____

Section A: HAVE YOU EVER HAD OR DO YOU HAVE?   Circle the correct response

1. High Blood Pressure _____ Yes/No
2. High Cholesterol/Triglycerides _____ Yes/No
3. Pain/tightness in the chest _____ Yes/No
4. Rheumatic Fever _____ Yes/No
5. Any Heart/Stroke condition _____ Yes/No
6. Gout _____ Yes/No
7. Stomach/Duodenal Ulcer _____ Yes/No
8. Liver/Kidney condition _____ Yes/No
9. Diabetes _____ Yes/No
10. Epilepsy _____ Yes/No
11. Are you a male 35 years or over, or a female 45 years or older? _____ Yes/No

Section B: DO YOU EXPERIENCE OR HAVE YOU EXPERIENCED?

1. A family history of heart disease, stroke or raised cholesterol of relatives
   under 65 years of age _____ Yes/No
2. Breathing difficulties or asthma _____ Yes/No
3. A Hernia _____ Yes/No
4. Arthritis _____ Yes/No
5. Back Pain _____ Yes/No
6. Muscular Pain/Cramps _____ Yes/No
7. Any major injuries _____ Yes/No
8. Do you smoke cigarettes/pipe/cigar _____ Yes/No
9. Are you on any prescribed medication? (describe) _____ Yes/No
10. Have you been hospitalised recently? (describe) _____ Yes/No
11. Do you have or have you had recently any infections or infectious diseases?
    (describe) _____ Yes/No
12. Are there any other conditions which may limit your activity program? _____ Yes/No

I represent and warrant to the Fitness Centre that I have furnished details of any medical
condition I have and of all recent medical treatment received by me.
I have read the foregoing and I understand it and any questions which may have occurred
to me have been answered to my satisfaction.

SIGNED: . . . .   DATE . . . .
            (Client)

WITNESS: . . . . DATE . . . .
            (Signature)   Please print name

Fig. 4.5: The Pre-Activity Questionnaire (NSW Fitness Council 1989)

Planning a Workout

Once all of the above factors are considered, emphasis needs to be given to the way in which an aerobic program should be carried out. All programs should consist of three essential parts: warm-up, conditioning and cool-down. Together these make up the *Three Segment Workout*.

The Warm-Up

A gentle warm-up should always precede strenuous activity. The purpose of this is:

• To stimulate the heart and lungs moderately and progressively
• To increase blood flow
• To increase body and muscle temperatures gradually
• To increase the metabolism of skeletal muscle
• To prevent muscle and joint injury
• To prepare the individual psychologically for the effect to follow.

A proper warm-up will consist of 2 parts:

1. General warm-up: This involves rhythmic movement of the entire body in order to increase circulation and body temperature. The time required will vary with the individual and the outside temperature. However, the commencement of sweating indicates that the body is ready for more vigorous activity.

2. Specific warm-up: This involves stretches and movements that are specifically used in the activities to follow. Specific warm-up should aid in the prevention of muscle strain. The actual skill to be used later should be performed at medium speed. Numerous examples of specific warm-up can be seen prior to sporting events. Examples of some warm-up stretches for various sports are shown in Figure 4.6. Other stretches are shown in Chapter 5.

The Conditioning Bout

The recommended activities for cardiovascular conditioning and weight control are those aerobic exercises listed in Table 4.1. These stimulate the cardiovascular system to induce a training effect. All exercise should be conducted according to the FITT plan.

The range of aerobic training regimes that can be used includes the following:

Jogging/Running

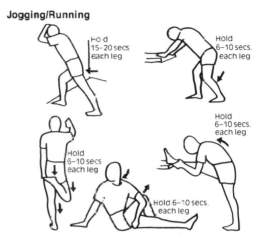

Football

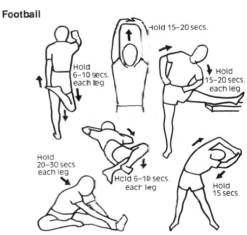

Tennis/Squash/Racquet Sports

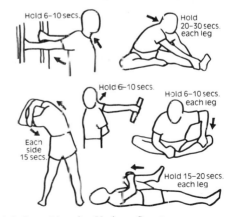

Fig. 4.6: Stretching for Various Sports

LSD (long slow distance) training is, as it would be expected, a system of slow steady exercise. It is perhaps the most common form of training and is particularly suitable for those with low initial fitness and older people (walking and jogging are good examples).

Interval training involves short bursts of intense activity interspersed with rest or recovery periods. For example, instead of jogging slowly over 5–10 miles, an athlete wishing to improve his/her anaerobic capacity as well as aerobic conditioning may run 10 × 400-metre laps at around three-quarter pace with 2–3 minute recovery periods between laps. This technique is not recommended for unfit individuals.

Calisthenics are exercises without weights using the body as resistance. To be aerobic they must be carried out continuously over the prescribed period. Examples are the 5BX, XBX and Canadian Air Force Fitness programs.

Circuit training can be carried out with or without weights. It consists of a series of exercises in sequence that are repeated in a given order. Exercises should be rotated so that all the major muscles of the body are stressed and no one muscle group is excessively fatigued.

The benefits of circuit training for the participant are:

• A compromise between aerobic and strength training
• Avoids problems of over-use
• Is good for balanced strength development
• Is not intimidating
• Is time-efficient
• Encourages group involvement
• Can be adapted easily for different ages and fitness levels

• Is not competitive
• Can be adapted to meet the needs of different sports
• Is a good weight loss exercise program
• Is an effective fitness program during rehabilitation
• Low injury risk.

The benefits of circuit training for the gym and instructor are:
• Suits a large cross section of the population
• Space efficient
• Easy and effective supervision
• Not physically demanding for the instructor
• Promotes a good gym atmosphere.

The Cool-Down

This is the tapering-off period. It is important to maintain the muscles' ability to return blood from the extremities to the heart. Following an exercise session a large supply of blood remains in the working muscles. If this is not returned promptly to the central circulation, pooling of the blood may occur in the muscles. If the brain doesn't receive sufficient blood fainting can occur.

Cooling down is best accomplished by a continuation of the activity at a lower intensity. Generally this involves keeping moving by walking or light jogging for some five minutes after exercise. Gentle movement should continue until the heart rate returns to a steady state. Static and PNF stretching should be included at the end of the cool-down. In fact, recent research suggests that greatest flexibility gains are achieved as a result of flexibility training following the exercise session.

Planning a Circuit Program

In simple terms circuit training is the arrangement of known and proven exercises designed to elicit maximum overall training effectiveness. Circuit training has as its objective the development of muscular and cardio-respiratory fitness. It aims at overall fitness rather than specific fitness for different activities.

Over the past few years circuit training has gained enormous popularity in fitness centres. The following could account for this:

1. It adds variety to an individual's training program
2. It does not discriminate between men and women

3. It is a good introduction for people wishing to commence a weight training program
4. It makes very efficient use of equipment
5. It accommodates different fitness levels
6. It adds a specific muscular endurance component to the training session
7. It incorporates all of the 3 S's of fitness.

Basically there are two ways of planning a circuit:
Method 1: This involves using fixed resistance, fixed repetitions and minimising the time taken to complete the circuit. 'Parcourse' programs in parks are examples of this method. The main advantage is that it is easy

to monitor improvement by recording the time taken to complete the circuit.

Method 2: In this case each exercise is carried out with a fixed resistance for as many repetitions as possible in a given period of time. The circuit class is an example of this method. The main advantage is that participants can work at their own pace without having to wait before stations. The use of the circuit timer will facilitate this method.

Exercise layout: The exercises in any circuit should be laid out in specific order to enhance the training effect and prevent overload of specific muscle groups. This can be done by:

• Alternating exercises to different body parts. For example a leg press can be followed by an arm curl; sit-ups followed by a leg curl.

• Using a large muscle activity between exercises which will increase the aerobic effect of the circuit. For example, running, cycling, mini-trampolining or step-ups.

Circuit training can be extremely demanding and beginners can very easily develop feelings of nausea and discomfort. As a result it is advisable that all beginners are:

• Adequately screened (see page 48)

• Taught the correct exercise technique

• Taught pulse taking and the concept of training heart rate range

• Warned against over-competitiveness

• Informed of the importance of warming up and cooling down.

Motivation and Participant Retention

Circuit training, like floor classes, should provide variety. Some of the techniques that can be used to provide this, and maintain participant interest, are:

• Using 'up-tempo' background music

• Varying the circuit sequence regularly

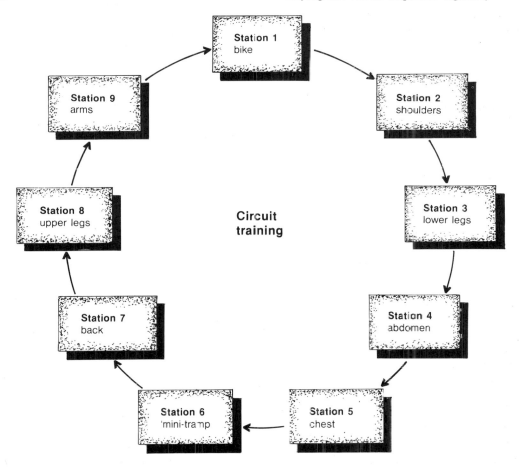

Fig. 4.7: Arrangement of an Aerobic Circuit

- Changing the direction of the circuit
- Varying the resistance for stronger individuals.

When designing a circuit there are three important variables that can be manipulated to alter the training emphasis of the program—the resistance, the set duration, and the rest duration.

Resistance: The amount of resistance will depend upon the equipment used, the desired training effect and the strength of participants.

Set Duration: The time allowed to perform each exercise can vary between 20 and 60 seconds to suit the fitness levels of participants and training objectives of the circuit.

Rest Duration: The recovery period between exercises can be increased or decreased to meet the desired training intensity. For example:

General conditioning	0–10 secs.
Strength and power	30–60 secs.
Older or very unfit	20–60 secs.

Other variables that can be manipulated in a circuit program are the duration of the circuit and the intensity at which each exercise is completed. Intensity can be monitored by recording heart rate (see page 43).

Following are two different types of circuit that are inexpensive and require little space. The first requires a few free weights and a timer. The second is even more basic and needs only a few sheets of paper, pencil and a bank of exercises.

Circuits Using Free Weights, Machines and Equipment

To ensure the circuit has an adequate aerobic component, exercises should be carried out with light weights and high repetitions (15–20), and preferably include the larger muscle groups.

Free Weight Circuit Examples of exercises for a free weight circuit incorporating some equipment are:

1. Squat
2. Bicep curl
3. Exercise bike
4. Bench press
5. Abdominal crunch
6. Power clean
7. Mini trampoline
8. Upright row
9. Abdominal crunch
10. Press behind neck
11. Exercise bike
12. Pullovers
13. Lunges
14. Dumbell flyes
15. Skipping

Machine System Equipment Circuit These circuits are becoming more popular with fitness centres establishing specific circuit rooms using a range of equipment. The machines systems used for circuits can be divided into two broad categories, those using hydraulic cylinders such as Hydra-Fitness and Titan and those using cams and cables such as Universal and Nautilus.

Fitness instructors should take into consideration the following when leading a machine circuit:

- Does all the equipment work properly?
- What level of resistance is the equipment set at?
- Does the equipment need to be wiped down after each person?
- Do all the participants know how to use each piece of apparatus?
- Do any of the participants have any limitations with regard to use of any of the equipment?

Circuit Using Floor Class Exercises

This type of circuit is a good substitute for an exercise class as it is done to music and most participants will be familiar with the exercises. Examples of exercise stations that can be used are:

1. Squats with lateral raise
2. Push-ups with hands wide
3. Shoulder lift (lie face down)
4. Abdominal crunch
5. Forward lunge
6. Side leg lifts (left side)
7. Push-ups from the knees with hands together
8. Reverse curl
9. Side leg lifts (right side)
10. Inner leg lifts (left leg)
11. Donkey kicks (right side)
12. Karate punches
13. Inner leg lifts (right side)
14. Donkey kicks (left side).

All the above exercises can be interspersed with aerobic movements such as running on the spot, skipping, travelling moves, push backs, etc.

Fitness instructors should take into consideration the following when designing and leading a circuit using floor class exercises:

- Do the participants know how to correctly execute each exercise?

- Does the circuit meet the right safety guidelines?
- Is the circuit well balanced to ensure all the major muscles are overloaded?
- Is there too much repetitive foot strike in the aerobic movements?
- Have the selected exercises been properly sequenced?

General Considerations for all Circuits

Space: Most circuits can be adapted to the allocated space. However, instructors should ensure that there is sufficient space between participants.

Music: The music selected must be motivational and should vary depending on the type of circuit.

Beginners: If possible give beginners some instruction on exercise technique before the circuit commences. Also, it is a good idea to place a beginner next to an experienced participant so that he/she can see how the exercise should be performed.

Length of time at each station: The ideal time per station is 30 seconds. However, it is important to encourage participants to move from one station to another as quickly as possible to get the greatest benefit from the allocated time.

Heart rate checks: As a general rule take a heart rate check after 15 minutes, at the end of the circuit and after the cool down.

Guidelines for Aerobic Exercise Programs

The following are suggested standards for conducting aerobic exercise programs:

1. The session must have a genuine aerobic component which lasts for a minimum of 20 minutes at an intensity measured preferably for a minimum heart rate of 120 bpm.

2. Participants should be encouraged to carry out such an exercise at least 3 times per week.

3. At least 5 minutes must be spent in slow stretching and warming up at the start of the program and in slow stretching and cooling down at the end.

4. Progression from warm-up to aerobic effort must be gradual as it should also be with cool-down.

5. Ballistic (bouncy) movements should be avoided as much as possible during the progression of the program, particularly for inexperienced exercisers.

6. As far as possible, classes should be structured to cater for beginner and advanced exercisers, with separate classes conducted for each.

7. All new participants in a class should be questioned as to their previous exercise levels and advised as to the level recommended for their purpose.

8. Attention must be given to the correct procedures in carrying out specific exercises.

9. Advice should be given to certain clients about the level of difficulty of some exercises (many men have difficulty with certain flexibility exercises more suited to women—adductor/abductor stretches, back flexes, etc.).

10. Advice should be given on the type of clothing to wear to prevent over-heating or chafing.

11. If classes are carried out to music, this should be such as to ensure a slow and gradual warm-up of at least 5 minutes and a similar cool-down.

12. Precautions must be taken at all times to prevent both acute and chronic injury. This includes the over-use of certain techniques such as bouncing on toes, or running with bare feet on hard surfaces.

13. Participants should be advised from the start of the program as to how long the exercise period will be and of any idiosyncracies in the program that may not be expected.

14. Participants must be asked if they are taking any form of medication, and if so, what this may be. Where no knowledge about a medication is immediately available, steps should be taken to ascertain contra-indications, if any.

15. Participants should be advised to exercise before rather than after eating; but limited fluid intake (with the exception of alcohol) before, and even during prolonged exercise, is advisable.

16. Special attention should be paid to the possibility of dehydration in hot weather.

17. All participants should be encouraged to wear well cushioned shoes in classes involving running, skipping or hopping.

18. Participants must never be permitted to join classes when they have not had sufficient warm-up.

5 Exercise Programming for Suppleness: Flexibility Training

Suppleness (flexibility) refers to the possible range of motion or movement of a joint or group of joints. Although this may be affected by structural damage to the bones of the joint, the most common factor affecting flexibility is the inability of the muscles surrounding a joint to stretch to an optimal length.

In most people, joints have the potential to move through a greater range of motion than the muscles that surround them will allow. Through regular stretching the muscles' capacity to extend fully is increased, thus allowing the joint a greater range of motion.

Flexibility is an important factor in all aspects of human movement, particularly sports-related activities. Many studies and observations show that more flexible athletes are better performers in their sport. Furthermore, limited flexibility results in restricted movement and a greater possibility of injury to the muscles.

Flexibility is improved by reduced muscle tension, using controlled force to increase the range of movement, and lengthening the connective tissue.

Why Stretch?

Without regular stretching, muscles tend to lose flexibility so that when called upon to perform an extreme movement, as in an emergency, they are less able to extend to their full range of movement, resulting in damage to the muscle tissue.

Certain sports are also responsible for a reduction in muscle flexibility. For example, jogging, football, hockey and boxing involve movements where muscles are not taken to their full range of stretch. This can lead to muscle tightness and shortening. Proper stretching even for short periods, daily, can help to:

1. **Prevent injuries:** Stretching improves the range of movement of a muscle. Hence, if a joint is stretched to its limit, a stretched muscle will allow greater movement.

2. **Improve biomechanical efficiency:** e.g. A tight Achilles tendon is inefficient because it does not allow a complete and strong push-off for each stride during running.

3. **Increase extensibility of muscles:** Increasing range of movement allows for greater speed and power in actions that require a wide range e.g. throwing in baseball, bowling in cricket.

4. **Improve co-ordination between muscle groups:** Where variability exists in opposing muscle groups weaknesses can develop in musculo-tendinous connections.

5. **Improve relaxation of muscles:** This is often an advantage for pre-competition warm-up, helping the athlete feel psychologically prepared for the action to follow.

6. **Decrease muscle tightening after movement:** Stretching after the event can diminish muscle tightening and prevent stiffness developing.

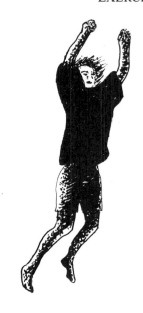

7. Counteract the possible restricting effects of hypertrophy training: For some sports, muscle bulking is desirable. But this can have the effect of shortening muscles that aren't put through their full range of movement. Stretching helps alleviate the problem.

Stretching helps to increase coordination between muscle groups

Factors Affecting Flexibility

A variety of factors can affect flexibility. These include:

Exercise: More active people tend to be more flexible.

Heat: An increase in temperature induced by either direct heat or the weather can increase the range of motion and elasticity of a muscle. Conversely, a decrease in temperature can result in a decrease in flexibility of as much as 20%. This accentuates the need for stretching before activities such as ice skating, skiing and swimming.

Age: Stiffness is often associated with advancing age. Muscle contractability remains, while elasticity is lost, resulting in tighter, stiffer muscles. A reduction in activity also decreases flexibility. Hence, increasing activity and muscle stretching can keep the effects of these changes to a minimum.

Warming Up: Warming up produces an increase in muscle temperature. The flexibility of joints and muscles is more easily achieved after an adequate warm-up period.

Sex: Most comparative studies have shown females to be more flexible than males in most joints, and to remain so throughout adult life. It is not known quite why this is so, but it has been attributed to the different training experiences of boys and girls early in life.

Specificity: Flexibility is specific to each joint and the angle of contraction of the muscles surrounding (or supporting) the joint. Hence flexibility programs should concentrate on those areas of the body that are to be involved in specific activity though the 'unused' muscles should not be neglected.

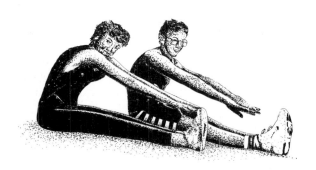

Females are generally more flexible than males and remain so throughout life.

Types of Stretching

Stretching exercises fall into 3 broad categories:

1. Passive stretching: sometimes referred to as **static stretching**. This form of stretching involves the gradual stretching of a muscle to a point where it is held, *without bouncing*, for 10 to 30 seconds. The muscle should be taken to a point where there is feeling in the muscle that it is being stretched. If the muscle is taken to the point of discomfort then the stretch should be eased off.

Static stretching is a safe and effective way of stretching muscles and connective tissue. Because it involves no sudden movements it does not provoke the stretch reflex as much as in ballistic stretching, and has a beneficial effect on the inverse stretch reflex.

Static stretching is best suited for:

• General stretching of all muscles
• The early stages of recovery from injury
• The cool-down phase following a vigorous exercise program.

2. Active stretching: sometimes referred to as **dynamic** or **range of movement stretching**. This form of stretching arose out of the concern that some people tend to over stretch in a passive or PNF situation. This may cause damage to the muscle and tendon fibres, particularly in the case of recovery from over-use injuries, such as tendinitis.

Range of movement (ROM) stretching has become an integral part of the warm up of most exercise classes to music. It involves the rhythmical movement of the major muscles that will be used in the exercise program. ROM stretches should be gentle repetitions of the types of movements that will be experienced in the workout.

Active stretching is best suited for:

• Stretching immediately before a period of vigorous activity (such as an exercise class to music)
• Stretching the muscle groups that cross the major joints (such as the shoulders, the hips, the knees and ankles).

3. Ballistic stretching: This form of stretching is bounce stretching, where the muscle is taken to its end of range of motion, and then over stretched by bouncing. This used to be the acceptable way of stretching, but has now been discarded because of a knowledge of the intra-muscular damage that may occur as a result of the 'stretch reflex'.

The stretch reflex: Muscle fibres contain sensory nerve endings called muscle spindles (see Chapter 2) whose main function is to send messages back from the muscle to inform about its state of stretch.

If the muscle is stretched, distortion of the central part of the muscle spindle causes the stretch reflex to automatically come into play to contract the muscle, thus avoiding damage through tearing.

The amount and rate of contraction elicited from the stretch reflex are proportional to the amount and rate of stretching. Hence, the faster and more forceful the stretch, the faster and more forceful the reflex contraction of the stretched muscle and thus the likelihood of the muscle tearing—particularly in an untrained muscle.

Bouncing, or 'ballistic' actions in exercise programs are therefore not recommended because of the potential damage caused by the stretch reflex. However, ballistic exercises may be important in the well-conditioned athlete who may require ballistic and explosive actions in his/her sport. But in this case actions should be preceded by either passive or active (ROM) stretching.

PNF Stretching

PNF stands for *Proprioceptive Neuromuscular Facilitation*. Although relatively recent in fitness training, PNF has been used in the rehabilitation of muscle and tendon injury for some time. A variation of this has now become the most accepted form of stretching for best results in flexibility training and injury prevention.

Research has shown that back flexion as measured by a sit-and-reach test can be improved by almost 200% over 3 months using PNF stretching as compared with static (slow) or ballistic (bouncing) stretching.

PNF involves a static stretch followed by an isometric contraction of a muscle against an immovable resistance (e.g. a partner). The muscle is then stretched further statically and the action repeated. Each isometric contraction is held for about 6 seconds (see Figure 5.1).

For PNF stretching the following precautions should be observed:

1. It should only be attempted after a total body warm-up.

2. The isometric contraction should never be explosive.

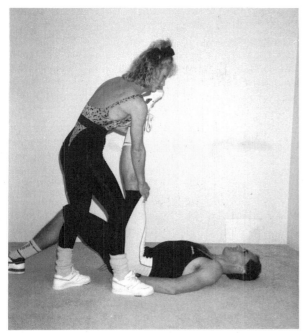

Fig. 5.1: *Hamstring stretch with partner.* Start by lying on the back and raising one leg and statically stretching it. Contract the hamstrings isometrically against the partner for 6 seconds. Relax them and statically stretch the hamstrings further and repeat the procedure.

3. A partner should provide only resistance in the isometric phase and *mild* assistance in the static stretch phase.

4. The isometric contraction should involve a gradual increase in effort in the first 2 seconds which is then sustained for an additional 4 seconds.

Why PNF Stretching Works

The PNF system is based on two fundamental principles:

1. A muscle can relax more fully after it has undergone a maximum isometric contraction and its resistance to stretching is therefore reduced.

2. A muscle becomes stronger if its antagonist is isometrically contracted immediately beforehand.

The preliminary isometric contraction makes the muscle more relaxed while it is being stretched. It also strengthens the contraction of the opposing muscles which are used to pull the body part into a more extreme stretch position.

PNF stretching was first developed by Herman Kabat in the 1940s and was primarily used for the rehabilitation of injured muscles. It has been suggested that it works through two processes:

1. 'Irradiation', or the spread of excitation through synergistic muscle contraction, and

2. 'Successive induction', which is the enhanced agonistic effort achieved after an antagonistic contraction.

Research on PNF stretching has been carried out by Dr Laurence Holt from Dalhousie University in Canada. Holt compared three stretching techniques: static, ballistic and PNF stretching in increasing trunk flexion in the seated position.

After 3 months, the average increase in range of motion for the slow, static method was 1.7 cm, for the ballistic method slightly less than 1.7 cm and for the PNF technique nearly 5 cm or almost 3 times greater than either of the other two methods.

PNF stretching is best done with a partner, although exercises can also be carried out individually (see Figure 5.2).

Overstretching is identified by a feeling of tension or mild pain that becomes greater the longer the stretch is held. Vibrating or quivering of the muscles also suggest overstretching.

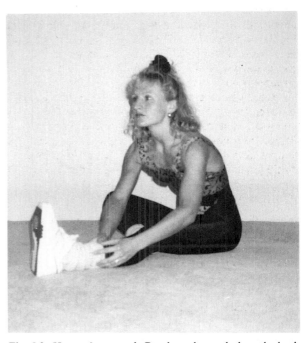

Fig. 5.2: *Hamstring stretch.* Bend one leg and place the heel close to the knee of the straight leg. With the back straight, reach towards the ankle with the hands. By holding the ankle and isometrically contracting the hamstrings and back muscles the stretch incorporates the PNF principles.

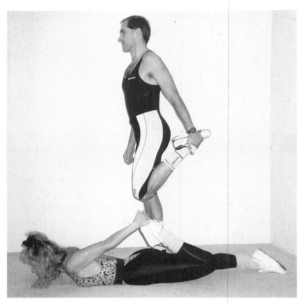

Fig. 5.3: *Quadricep stretch.* While standing or lying down pull the heel of the bent leg into the buttock. When doing this stretch it is important to keep the knees together. Again, this stretch can incorporate the PNF principles.

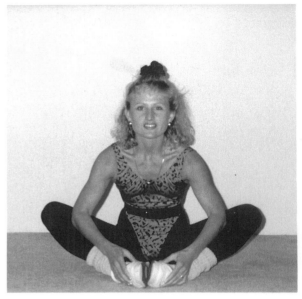

Fig. 5.4: *Adductor stretch.* Start by placing the heels together and resting the elbows on the knees. Exert pressure on the knees with the elbows for 6 seconds. Relax, then repeat the procedure with the knees wider apart.

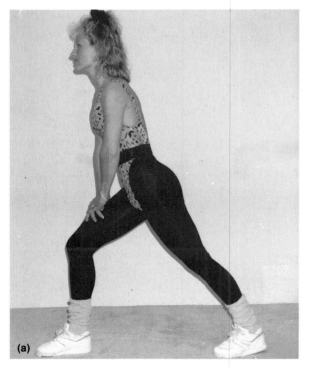

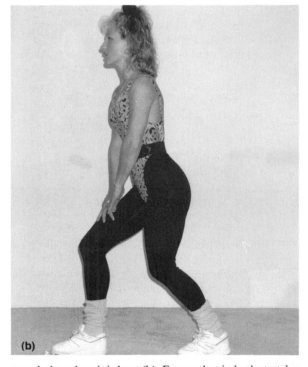

Fig. 5.5: *Calf stretch.* When stretching the calf both the gastrocnemius and soleus muscles should be stretched. To stretch the gastrocnemius the back leg is straight (a) and to stretch the soleus it is bent (b). Ensure that in both stretches the upper body weight is taken on the front leg.

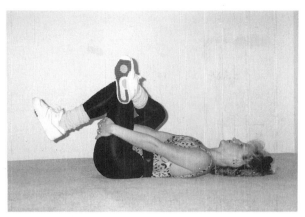

Fig. 5.6: *Gluteal stretch.* Pull the leg towards the chest. Incorporate a PNF stretch by contracting the held leg for 6 seconds, then relaxing and repeating.

Developmental Stretch

A developmental stretch should follow an easy stretch. In this case the tension of the stretch is increased to a level just beyond the easy stretch. The increased distance is determined by the tension felt, and not by a specific goal.

This stretch should again be held for at least 10 seconds, thereby allowing muscle fibres to stretch out slowly and stay stretched for a period of time. In the proper developmental stretch, the feeling of the stretch should decrease the longer the stretch is held, as it did with the easy stretch.

A Warning on Stretching

It should be pointed out that the field of flexibility training has only recently attracted the interest of researchers, hence there is much to learn. Meanwhile, not all authorities accept the value of stretching.

For example, US sports medicine physician Richard H. Dominguez, author of the *Complete Book of Sports Medicine*, claims stretching before exercise can cause rather than prevent injury.

According to Dominguez, runners in particular may over-stretch muscles and tendons beyond a point of active control. This could cause muscle fibre damage where prior problems exist in knees or joints. Instead of excessive static stretching, Dominguez favours a warm-up of a gentle range of motion exercises starting gradually and building up.

Critics of the Dominguez view claim that although it has some merit, it can be over-generalised. In exercise like gymnastics or floor classes where range of motion demands are great, gentle stretching as well as a general warm-up is necessary.

Specific Flexibility Tests

The following 5 flexibility tests require no equipment and can be used to assess flexibility on a group basis such as an exercise class to music.

Test 1: Sit and Reach

This is a general flexibility test for the lower back and hamstring muscle groups. Adequate flexibility in the back and hamstrings is considered very important for the prevention of lower back pain. The lower back and hamstrings are very common sites of tightness in the general population as well as in some groups of athletes. Because of its simplicity and quickness, the sit and reach test is the single most commonly used test for flexibility in fitness evaluations.

Procedure
• Sit on the floor with the legs out straight

• Place the soles of the feet against a flat board
• With the legs straight bend forward at the hips
• Reach forward and with the hands try to touch the toes and then stretch past the toes.

Goals
• Not touching the toes is poor
• Touching the toes is average
• Reaching a hand length beyond the toes is very good
• Reaching up to the middle of the forearm is excellent.

For more detailed comparison tables for the sit and reach test see Chapter 10.

Test 2: Hamstring Test

The sit and reach test is a good overall flexibility test that measures the range of movement of a number of joints. The following hamstring test specifically measures the suppleness of the hamstring muscles reflected by the maximum possible angle of hip flexion.

Procedure
• Lie on the back with both legs out straight
• Keep the lower back flat and raise one leg to the vertical position
• A partner can stabilise the raised leg and gently push the leg to maximum hip flexion.

Goals
• Less than 90 degrees at the hip is poor
• 90 degrees at the hip is acceptable
• 105 degrees at the hip is good.

Test 3: Quadricep Test

The quadricep muscle group is a hip flexor and plays an important role in correct pelvic alignment. In addition adequate quadricep flexibility reduces the risk of knee cap problems such as chrondromalacia patellar and patellar tendinitis.

Procedure
• Lie on the stomach with both legs out straight
• Bend one knee so that the heel of the foot is close to the buttocks
• Contract the abdominals to keep the hips on the floor
• Have a partner gently push the ankle towards the buttocks.

Goals
• Heel cannot touch the buttock is poor
• Heel touches the buttock is average
• Heel touches the buttock with no resistance is good.

Test 4: Shoulder Extension Test

Adequate shoulder extensor flexibility is very important for allowing correct biomechanics when the arms are used in an overhead position. Inadequate flexibility can potentially contribute to shoulder injury as well as compensatory upper back injury.

Procedure
• Sit on the floor with the knees comfortably bent
• Bring the arm (straight) forward and fully overhead
• Throughout the movement contract the abdominals to prevent the back from arching or rotating
• A partner can gently push the back to its maximum range of movement.

Goals
• Straight arm in front of the shoulder is poor
• Straight arm in line with the shoulder and hip is good
• Straight arm behind the shoulder is good.

Rules for Stretching

The following are basic principles which should be followed in any program involving stretching:

• Breathe slowly, deeply and evenly
• Do not stretch to the point where breathing is strained
• Do not over stretch. Go to the point where the stretch is felt but no pain
• Hold the stretch in a comfortable position; tension should subside as the stretch is held
• Stretch only when the muscles are warm
• Concentrate on relaxing the area being stretched
• If appropriate, combine different types of stretching in one session. Avoid ballistic or bouncy stretching
• Stretch before and after an extended exercise period
• Hold static stretches for 15 to 30 seconds and if possible even longer.

Guidelines for Flexibility Training

The following are tips for flexibility training based on some of the limited research evidence available:

1. Bouncy, jerky movements should be avoided. These can be potentially hazardous, particularly with untrained muscles.

2. Stretching should progress from major joints to more specific joints. This ensures adequate support for all muscle groups involved.

3. Stretching should be carried out immediately before, after and even during an active sports event. Research

has shown that up to one third of the flexibility gains from stretching can be lost in half an hour of sitting still before competition, and up to two-thirds in an hour.

4. Sport-specific flexibility should be developed by identifying the movements of the sport and training specifically in these movements.

5. Flexibility training should be regular, i.e. 3–4 times a week. Noticeable increases in flexibility with training can be achieved within 2–3 weeks. Decreases can occur almost as quickly.

6. If stretching is discontinued as a result of injury, qualified advice should be sought before flexibility training is recommenced.

7. Stretching involving hyperextension of the lower back can often aggravate minor injuries and therefore should involve special care and attention, particularly with inexperienced exercisers.

8. Pregnant women should only undertake flexibility training under supervision. During pregnancy, hormones are released which soften ligaments to make the skeletal structures of the hips and pelvis extensible for carrying an infant. This increases the hypermobility of joints, but exercises that place strain on these hypermobile joints can cause pain and chronic joint problems.

9. With PNF stretching, careful attention should be paid to the correct execution of exercises. If this is not done, the results could be counter-productive.

10. The optimal time for holding an isometric contraction in a PNF stretch is 6 seconds. Other static stretching can be held from 15–30 seconds.

6 Exercise Programming for Strength: Resistance Training

Weight training or resistance training is traditionally viewed by the community as a pastime for body-builders and strength athletes who wish to 'pump iron' to increase muscle size. For fitness instructors the area of resistance training is more far reaching than this view. For example, an exercise class to music is a form of resistance training where body weight is the resistance. More recently 'The New Body Class', which incorporates dumbells into the aerobic tracks, uses the weight training principle of light weights with many repetitions to improve muscular endurance.

Resistance training has gained acceptance with a variety of people, from the distance runner who lifts weights to maintain some upper body development to women wanting a change from the exercise to music class.

The Benefits of Weight Resistance Training

There are many positive benefits of weight training. Some of these are listed below.

Weight training can:

i)   Improve aerobic conditioning through circuit training
ii) Be structured to develop muscular strength, speed and power
iii) Make significant changes in body composition
iv) Improve posture
v)   Increase lean body tissue (muscle bulk)
vi) Be structured to strengthen muscles for sports performance
vii) Be used to rehabilitate muscles following injury
viii) Improve an individual's self esteem
ix) Be adapted to all fitness levels
x)   Increase metabolic rate to help decrease body fat.

Weight Training Terminology

Resistance training programs will vary according to the specific requirement of the program. Variations in general are based on:

1. Repetitions (reps), or the number of times an exercise movement is repeated without a rest.

2. Sets, or the number of groups of repetitions of an exercise.

3. Resistance (load), or the amount of weight used in an exercise.

4. Repetition maximum, or the maximum number of

repetitions that can be completed with a given resistance (e.g. a 10 RM is performed when only 10 repetitions can be completed not 9 or 11). Hence the greater the number of RM the lighter is the weight that can be lifted. The development of a particular feature of muscle performance is directly related to the load used (e.g. for strength 6 RM should be used, whereas for muscular endurance 15 RM should be used). Some exercises require care in using RM loading due to

possible injury. A classic example is the military press which can place enormous stress on the lower back if the correct technique is not used.

5. Rest is necessary for the regrowth of muscle tissue after overload. Also, rest periods are dependent on the energy systems the person wishes to stress and the specific purpose for which the training is being undertaken.

Uses of Resistance Training

Resistance training can be used for one or more of the following purposes:

i) *To increase strength*. Strength is the ability to exert force.
ii) *To improve power*. Power is the ability to exert force in a short period of time.
iii) *To add lean body tissue*. This refers to the hypertrophy of muscle to increase size. Often referred to as muscle bulk.
iv) *To improve muscular endurance*. This refers to the capacity of a muscle or muscle group to keep contracting efficiently over extended periods of time.

The resistance training regimes for strength, power, lean body mass and muscular endurance are summarised in Table 6.1. In certain circumstances a

combination of these can be carried out i.e. strength and muscle endurance.

Table 6.1: Resistance Training Regimes

Purpose	Weight	Reps	Sets	Ex. speed	Rest
Strength	2RM–6RM (advanced)	2–6	3–6	slow/med	3–5 min
	8RM–12RM (beginner)	8–12	2–3	slow/med	2–3 min
Power	med/heavy	4–6	3–6	fast/max explosive	3–5 min
Muscle endurance	15+ RM	15–30	2–3	med	minimal
Lean body mass	med/heavy	6–20	3–5	slow/med	1–2 min

Forms of Resistance Training

There are three general forms of resistance training. These are constant resistance, variable resistance and accommodating resistance.

Constant Resistance

When using constant resistance equipment, the level of effort changes throughout the range of motion. As the lever varies, the weight lifted either feels heavier (sometimes referred to as the sticking point) or lighter depending on the position of the joint. The difficulty in overcoming the resistance varies with the joint angle, an example being the bicep curl (see Figure 6.1). It is easier to curl the bar at the beginning and end of the

movement than the mid portion. Some examples of this form of training include free weights (barbells and dumbells), the lifter's own body weight (chins and dips) and some of the older style pin loaded weight machines.

Variable Resistance

Variable resistance equipment compensates for the leverage changes in a joint's range of motion. This equipment relates the body's leverage with the machine, thereby allowing the maximum intensity to be placed on the muscles over the complete range of motion. Variable resistance equipment imposes an increasing

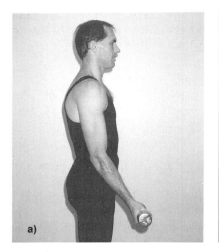
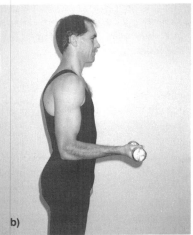
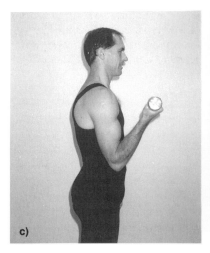

Fig. 6.1: The Bicep Curl a) strong commencement phase b) weak mid phase c) strong conclusion phase

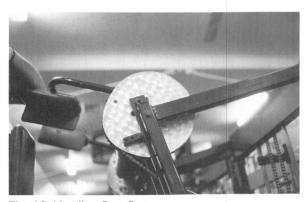

Fig. 6.2: Nautilus Cam System

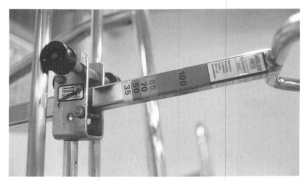

Fig. 6.3: Universal Rolling Levers

Table 6.2: The Effectiveness of the Different Systems

RATING THE EFFECTS OF EQUIPMENT TYPES ON SELECTED TRAINING GOALS ON A SCALE OF 1 TO 10)	Dumbells & Barbells	Constant Resistance Machines	Cam Machines	Lever Machines	Hydraulic Machines	Clutch & Flywheel Machines
Muscular size increases	10	8	7	7	5	5
Muscular strength increases	10	5	6	6	8	7
Explosive power increases	9	5	5	5	10	10
Sport skills carryover for the movement employed	9	5	5	5	5	8
Sport skills carryover for the velocity/acceleration employed	9	5	3	5	7	7
Quality of overload through the entire exercise set	6	6	7	7	9	8
Quality of muscular isolation	10	8	8	8	8	9
Overall versatility	10	6	5	6	5	9
TOTAL EFFECTIVENESS SCORE	73	48	46	49	57	63
	constant resistance		variable resistance		accommodating resistance	

load throughout the range of movement of the joint. This is accomplished through changing the relationship of the fulcrum and the lever arm in the weight machine as the exercise progresses. Nautilus use a cam and pulley system (Figure 6.2), while Universal use rolling levers to achieve this result (Figure 6.3).

Accommodating Resistance

By controlling the speed of movement, it is possible to considerably improve the overload through the entire range of movement. This is done by using hydraulic systems (Figure 6.4), air systems and clutch plates in tandem with flywheels. The new accommodating resistance devices allow maximum force to be applied against the resistance through the entire range of motion. Most of these accommodating resistance devices can also be adjusted to infinite gradations of speed ranging from very fast to very slow.

Types of Muscle Contraction

There are three main types of muscle contraction of interest to the weight trainer:

1. Isometric Training

The term isometric comes from the Greek *isometrikos* meaning literally 'the same length' or 'no change in length'. Isometric (or static) exercises are those done where a muscle develops tension without changing length. In fact, the muscle does shorten internally during an isometric contraction, but this is countered by a contraction of the antagonist muscle or the resistance of an immovable object.

Isometrics are useful for developing strength in weak spots and for increasing strength and preventing injury at the limits of the range of motion. Isometrics are particularly useful for sports such as downhill skiing, judo, gymnastics and windsurfing, where a position may have to be held for some time.

Although isometric training received quite a deal of attention in the 1950s and 1960s it is rarely practised today unless it is included with other weight training techniques. Strength increases associated with isometric training are specific to the joint angle at which the training is performed, and so for a full range of motion training effect to occur, this training would have to incorporate the unlimited range of joint angles. Even then the static nature of the training would have little benefit for the dynamic nature of most sports.

Some problems associated with isometric training include: minimal training of the neuro-muscular system; progress is difficult to assess and hence motivation to keep training may be hard to attain; and isometric contractions produce significantly higher systolic and diastolic blood pressures.

Functional isometric training for various sports can be carried out using weights or movable resistance where an isometric contraction is combined with an isotonic movement. For example, Pyke (1980) has pointed out that the following exercises with weights can be made isometric by holding the resistance at the joint angle specified:

Exercise	Joint angle
Bench press	Elbow joint at 90°
Arm curls	Elbow joint at 90°
Heel raises	Foot at 135°
Dead lift	Knee joint at 135°

2. Isotonic Training

The term isotonic literally means of equal tension. It implies that the muscle develops a certain tension or

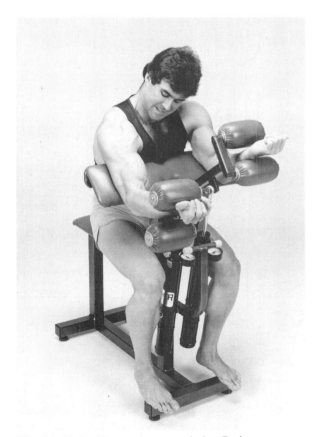

Fig. 6.4: Hydra-Fitness Accommodating Resistance

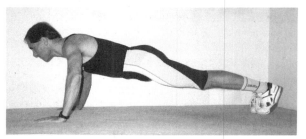

Fig. 6.5: The Push-up a) The upward phase—concentric

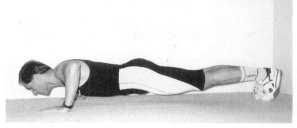

b) The downward phase—eccentric

force in lifting and lowering a load. In fact, the force developed by the muscle is variable depending on the lever at the joint.

There are two types of isotonic contractions. These are known as concentric and eccentric contractions.

i) **A concentric contraction** is often referred to as a positive contraction. It is a contraction where the muscle develops tension when shortening. For example, the upward phase of the bicep curl (the bicep is shortening) is a concentric contraction.

ii) **An eccentric contraction** is often referred to as a negative contraction. It is a contraction where the muscle develops tension while lengthening. For example, the downward phase of the bicep curl (the bicep is lengthening) is an eccentric contraction. A simple way of working out the eccentric phase is as follows: the eccentric phase occurs when the muscle is acting as a brake against the force of gravity, i.e. when lowering a weight.

In the push-up exercise the triceps and pectorals contract eccentrically in the descent phase and then contract concentrically to bring the person back to the starting position (Figure 6.5).

In order to get the greatest benefit out of the eccentric contraction the muscle must work against gravity. This means that the slower the eccentric contraction the greater the tension developed. As a general rule the eccentric phase should take twice as long as the concentric phase, i.e. if the concentric phase takes 2 seconds the eccentric should take 4 seconds.

Isotonic training with weights was developed in the late 1940s using the concept of Repetition Maximum (RM) for determining the amount of weight used. An RM is defined as the maximal load a muscle or muscle group can lift a given number of times before fatiguing.

For years it has been thought that strength could be improved only by using heavy resistance with low repetitions, and endurance by using light resistance with high repetitions. Recent studies have shown, however, that there is a good deal of carry-over from one type of training to another, even though the basic principle may still apply.

3. Isokinetic Training

An isokinetic contraction is one in which maximal tension is developed throughout the full range of movement. This requires special equipment in which

Table 6.1: Summary of advantages and disadvantages of the three most common types of resistance training programs

Criterion	Comparative rating		
	Isokinetic	Isometric	Isotonic
Rate of strength gain	Excellent	Poor	Good
Rate of endurance gain	Excellent	Poor	Good
Strength gain over range of motion	Excellent	Poor	Good
Time per training session	Good	Excellent	Poor
Expense	Poor	Excellent	Good
Ease of performance	Good	Excellent	Poor
Ease of progress assessment	Poor	Good	Excellent
Adaptability to specific movement patterns	Excellent	Poor	Good
Least possibility of muscle soreness	Excellent	Good	Poor
Least possibility of injury	Excellent	Good	Poor
Skill improvement	Excellent	Poor	Good

(From E. Fox, 1979)

speed of the movement is kept constant over the full range of the movement regardless of the tension applied. Hence, if the movement is made as fast as possible, the tension generated by the muscle will be maximal throughout the full range of motion.

Isokinetic training is relatively new and has therefore not yet been extensively evaluated scientifically. Research that has been carried out has shown significant strength gains. But in comparison with other isotonic devices the gains are relative to the type of equipment used for evaluation. For example,

athletes trained on isokinetic machines develop greater increases in strength than athletes trained isotonically, if the measure of strength is isokinetic. If the measure is isotonic, the opposite is true.

Isokinetic training is particularly useful in the rehabilitation of injury and in sports training which requires maximal power output throughout the full range of a muscle contraction. Furthermore, because isokinetic contractions can be made at speed, this type of training can assist in power and speed for various sporting activities.

Modern Resistance Training Modalities

Water Resistance Equipment (Triton)

The person using this equipment depresses a tiny switch which is fitted to the index finger. The switch activates a pump which increases the level of weight. The switch is then released, allowing the water (weight) to flow back to its source at a smooth, precise rate. The resistance allows the exerciser to continuously modify the weight used during each exercise so that each repetition is performed with maximum resistance (e.g. each repetition is the momentary 1 RM).

Hydraulic Equipment (Hydra-Fitness)

Hydraulic equipment varies both the resistance and the speed of movement throughout the range of motion. This system, using hydraulic cylinders, incorporates both isotonic and isokinetic principles. The manufacturers of Hydra-Fitness equipment refer to this combination as Powernetics (Figure 6.6). The cylinders have a 1–6 setting allowing for a change in resistance. A setting of 1 allows for a large aperture between the cylinders which provides light resistance. Conversely

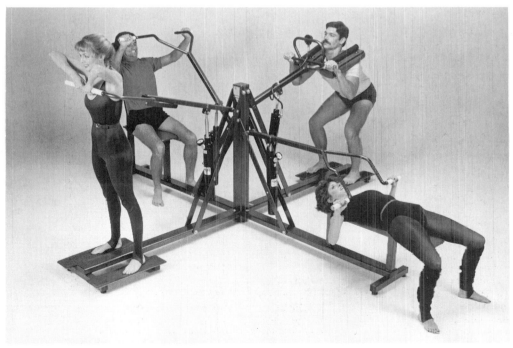

Fig. 6.6: Multi-
Station
Hydra-Fitness

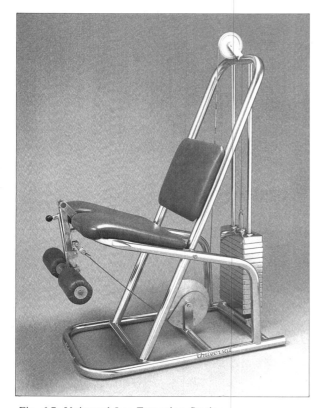

Fig. 6.7: Universal Leg Extension Station

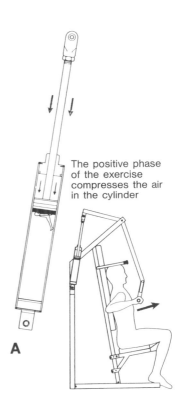

The positive phase of the exercise compresses the air in the cylinder

A

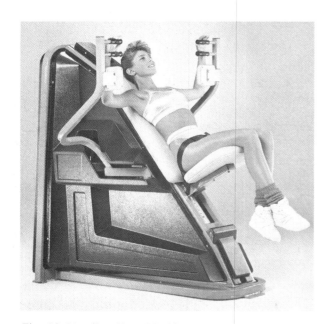

Fig. 6.8: Nautilus Chest Machine

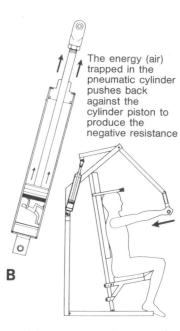

The energy (air) trapped in the pneumatic cylinder pushes back against the cylinder piston to produce the negative resistance

B

Fig. 6.9: Keiser a) The positive or concentric contraction
b) The negative or eccentric contraction

a setting of 6 allows for a small aperture resulting in a greater resistance. As a result of the hydraulic cylinders, Hydra-Fitness provides the lifter with a double concentric movement, allowing for two antagonistic movements to be completed using one piece of equipment (there are minimal eccentric contractions when using Hydra-Fitness equipment).

Dynamic Variable Resistance (DVR) Isotonic (Universal)

Consists of a variety of pin loaded weight stations designed using pulleys and guide rails. Universal's DVR (Figure 6.7) varies resistance to coincide with either the improving biomechanical advantage or with the muscles' decreased leverage to ensure maximum muscular effort throughout the full range of movement. A visual scale on the lever arm shows the percentage of increase of resistance driving the lifting stroke.

Variable Resistance Isotonic (Nautilus)

The heart of the Nautilus system is the cam, which is an 'off-round' wheel with a non-central axis of rotation shaped like a nautilus shell.

The radius of the nautilus cam changes as it turns. This acts to automatically vary the load to accommodate the weak and strong phases of the lifting stroke (Figure 6.8).

Air Pressure (Keiser Cam 2)

Pressurised pneumatic cylinders with compressed air create the resistance in this system. A pressure regulator located within easy reach of the trainee is used to vary air pressure so that either each repetition is a maximal force output or a set speed of performance is attained for each rep. This system allows for both concentric and eccentric contraction over the full range of movement. As air is compressed within the cylinder its pressure increases, thus increasing the force output on the cylinder.

Modern Techniques of Overload

The progressive overload principle is one of the most fundamental and important principles of muscle physiology. It states that to elicit improvements in muscle size, strength or endurance, the muscle must be placed under stress levels greater than it was previously used to and in a way specific to the required physiological outcomes. This can be achieved by either:

• Increasing the resistance or weight load
• Increasing the number of repetitions
• Increasing the speed of contraction
• Increasing the duration of the workout (sets, exercises)
• Decreasing the rest periods (up to a point) between sets.

More esoteric overloading techniques sometimes based on unclear physiological principles have been used for years, particularly by bodybuilders and sports trainers. In fact, this is one aspect of resistance training where the practice has often preceded the theory.

It is clear also that individuality has to be taken into consideration in evaluating overloading practices. Where some individuals respond well to some over-loading techniques, others do less well. Hence it is important for the fitness instructor to know the range of techniques available. The following is a list of overload techniques gathered from sports training and bodybuilding practices.

1. Blitzing This is the practice of bombarding a muscle or muscle group on any one training day. This can take the form of several exercises aimed at working the muscle from different angles.

2. Forced repetitions These require a partner or 'spotter' such that assistance can be given in that part of the movement where biomechanical advantage is least, and hence where the muscle is weakest. This then means a heavier weight can be lifted through the full range of movement.

For example, in the arm curl motion a 'sticking point' is reached about where the elbows are at right angles. If assistance is given through this point, a heavier weight can be used through the full range of motion.

When spotting a lifter, whether it be for forced reps or just during a normal set, the spotter should:

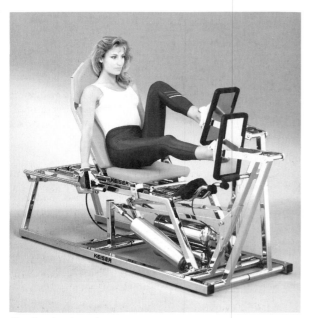

Overload using air pressure

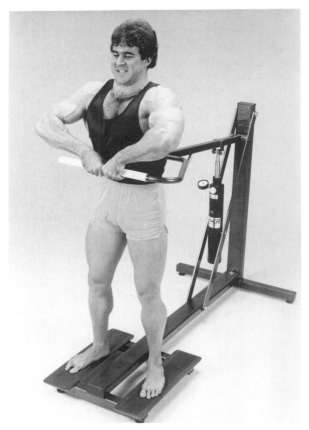

Overload using hydraulic cylinders

- Concentrate throughout the lift
- Check the bar is loaded correctly
- Check for weights sliding loose
- Determine what signals to use
- Determine how many reps are to be attempted
- Always check the lifter's form
- Encourage the lifter.

3. Cheating This is a technique only recommended for experienced weight trainers where auxiliary muscles are used to assist a prime mover in a movement. For example, in arm curls the trunk is bent forward slightly enabling the contraction of the back muscles to assist the lifter to lift a heavier weight through the weakest point of the movement. This means a heavier weight can be used and the muscle is thus overloaded through the strong phases of the movement.

Remember, when cheating, use gentle body motions to assist lifting the weight to the finished position. Never snap the weight through its range of motion.

4. Negative repetitions These capitalise on the fact that strength and bulk improvements in muscle are aided by exaggerated eccentric (lowering) contractions of the muscle. In a negative repetition the weight is only lowered enabling more weight to be used to over stress the muscle eccentrically. Spotters are generally required to lift the weight for the lifter so that it can then be lowered.

An example of negative repetitions would be where the weight is lowered to the chest slowly in the bench press and then returned to the rack by the spotters so the action can be repeated. Eccentric contractions are thought to place greater stress on muscle tissue than concentric actions because of the negative use of gravity in the former.

5. Pre-exhaustion This is where a muscle is isolated in an exercise and fatigued before being co-opted for further work in a compound exercise which immediately follows. The second or compound exercise enables the muscle previously exhausted to continue working because it is aided by synergists.

An example of a complete pre-exhaust workout is as follows:

Shoulders   Dumbell lateral raise
             Press behind neck

Chest	Dumbell flyes
	Bench press
Thighs	Leg extension
	Squats
Back	Lat pulldown
	Seated row
Biceps	Preacher curl
	Narrow grip chin up
Triceps	Pressdown
	Dips

6. Rest pause This is a technique practised by body-builders for increasing intensity of effort. It is done by overloading a muscle such that only 1 RM can be carried out and a pause is necessary (perhaps 10 seconds) before it can be done again and again, over a set number of repetitions.

This is a high-intensity technique that should be carried out only by experienced lifters.

7. Up and down the rack This is a principle similar to pyramiding, except that weights from light to heavy gradations are arranged on a weight rack and exercises carried out with each of these, with weight increasing and then decreasing, until exhaustion.

8. Pyramid training This refers to the practice of increasing resistance step by step over sets or repetitions. It allows the person to start easily, build up to a peak and then taper off. The resistance is increased step by step over a number of sets then the load is decreased when the peak is reached (Table 6.3).

Table 6.3: The Squat Workout—Pyramid Style

Sets	Weight	Reps
1	50 kg	20
2	60 kg	12
3	65 kg	8
4	75 kg	4
5	60 kg	max
6	50 kg	max

9. Compound training (super-sets, tri-sets, giant sets) These are training methods which combine exercises for the same or antagonist body part without a rest between the exercises.

• *Super-sets* a) antagonist e.g. a leg extension followed by a leg curl, or b) same body part e.g. a bench press followed by dumbell flyes.

• *Tri-sets* for the same body part e.g. the deltoids using the following exercises:

Dumbell bent over raises
Press behind neck
Dumbell lateral raises.

• *Giant sets* which are super-sets with more than 2 exercises carried out without rest in between. Giant sets for the same body part e.g. the chest, using bench press followed by:

'Pec' dec
Incline dumbell press
Dumbell flyes.

10. Hybrid exercise/compound repetitions This method involves the use of several joints of the body moving through a greater range of motion than is normal with single exercises. Thus, instead of carrying out three or four exercises in a circuit, they can all be done in the one repetition. For example, the power clean could be followed by a front squat, then a push press, then an overhead squat, then finish by lowering the bar to chest and placing it on the ground.

11. Triple drop For many years, bodybuilders and other athletes have used the method of dropping or reducing the level of resistance (weight) during a set of repetitions to work a muscle area as thoroughly as possible. This is done by choosing a weight on a barbell, dumbell or machine that permits the user to perform only three or four repetitions. When failure is achieved, assistants remove only enough weight (usually 10%) to allow continuation of the exercise for another three or four repetitions. This procedure is repeated three times or until the muscle group is worked to a point of complete failure.

Steps to Consider in Resistance Training Programming

The steps involved in developing resistance training programs are:

1. Determine goals
2. Select training regime
3. Select exercises
4. Select training method
5. Select techniques of overload
6. Teach correct form
7. Evaluate progress.

Tips on Designing Weight Training Programs

1. Building lean body mass for beginners

- Use a moderate weight i.e. 8–12 RM
- Select one isolation and one compound exercise per body part. For example for the chest select the 'pec dec' followed by the bench press.
- Perform 2–3 sets of the 8–12 RM for each exericse in every workout. When more than 12 reps can be completed in the final set increase the weight used 2½ to 5%. Initially only use 1 set of each exercise for the first 2–4 weeks.
- Exercise three days per week with a rest day in between each workout.

2. Building lean body mass for intermediate to advanced

- Vary the load of the weights used. For example, alternate one heavy session of 4–6 RM with a medium session of 8–12 RM. These sessions should be alternated in a split workout (4 days a week).
- Increase the number of exercises to work the muscles from a variety of angles.
- Increase the total number of sets (4–5) per exercise.

3. Developing a strength training program

- Most authorities suggest that the resistance used should be greater than 80% of 1 RM.
- Use around 3–6 sets of less than 6 repetitions.
- Use mostly compound movements and select 3–4 exercises per body part.
- Where possible incorporate periodisation into the strength program
- Use a wide variety of exercises when programming for sport.

Russian training authorities suggest the following program to increase strength after a general warm-up is performed:

Load	90–95% of 1 RM
Reps	2–3
Sets	2–3
Rest	9–10 secs between reps
	4–6 mins between sets

This style of training can only be maintained for periods of about 6 weeks and is often interspersed with a muscle hypertrophy program such as:

Load	75–80% of 1 RM
Reps	8–12
Sets	2–3
Rest	1½–2 mins between sets

Instructors should note the above strength programs are only recommended for experienced resistance trainers.

4. Developing speed or explosive strength

Explosive strength can be developed by moving a heavy external resistance as quickly as possible. The percentage of the 1 RM used is often the determining factor in programming for these two categories.

An example of a speed/strength program is as follows:

Load	30–70% 1 RM
Reps	6–8 with high velocity
Sets	2–3 repeated 2–3 times
Rest	9–10 secs between reps
	4–6 mins between sets
	8–10 mins between sequences

Plyometrics

In recent years reactive training, commonly called plyometrics, has come into vogue to develop explosive speed. Plyometrics refers to specific exercises which encompass a rapid stretching of the muscles that are undergoing eccentric stress. This is followed by a rapid concentric contraction of the same muscles.

The most common plyometrics exercise is the depth jump where the person stands on a box approximately 1 metre high, then jumps off the box and lands on the balls of the feet. This is followed by an explosive vertical jump. To develop optimal speed and strength the time on the ground should be minimal: if too long is spent on the ground the eccentric tension developed will be lost into the ground instead of being converted to concentric force (see Figure 6.10).

Plyometric exercises can be planned using: jumps, medicine ball throws, handstand jumps and clap push-ups. In fact the limiting factor to developing plyometric exercises is the instructor's imagination.

5. Developing muscular endurance

Muscular endurance refers to tolerance against fatigue following high repetition work. The aim in training for muscular endurance is to maintain somewhat higher tension in the muscles than they are normally accustomed to.

Circuit training is an ideal method of training muscular endurance (see Chapter 4) as the

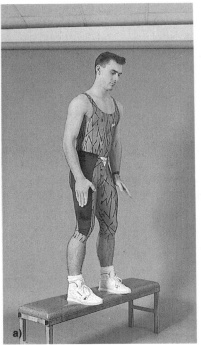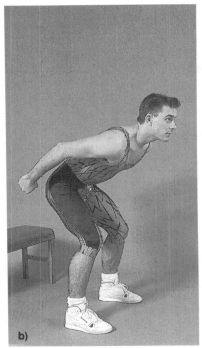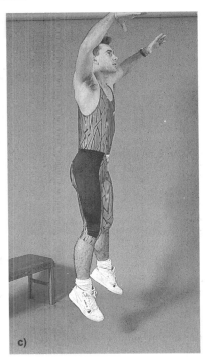

Fig. 6.10: The Depth Jump

manipulation of the load and rest periods can be adapted to specific needs of each individual.

6. Toning program
The basic guidelines for developing a toning program are as follows:

- light to moderate weight
- 1-2 sets per exercise
- 2-3 exercises per body part
- use mainly compound movements
- use a circuit structure
- program 3 sessions per week.

7. Circuit training with weights
Research on the energy expenditure involved in traditional weight training programs suggests that this is usually insufficient to produce an aerobic effect. Although individual exercises may be strenuous, the amount of time devoted to the exercises *per se* is usually short. The rate of oxygen consumed has been estimated to be roughly the equivalent of walking at 4 mile per hour pace, gardening or swimming at a slow speed. This means that such exercise would be of little value as the major component of a weight control or cardiovascular conditioning program.

It is possible to achieve aerobic benefit by combining exercises with weights in an aerobic circuit (see Chapter 4). In the fitness centre this can be done either on an individual or group basis, using traditional free weights or the modern weight training systems mentioned above.

Variation in Training

If training is to be adhered to over an extended period of time there needs to be some variety in the training stimulus. Over the last few years the concept of periodisation has become widely accepted as a way of varying both the volume and the intensity of training over a period of time to reach specific training goals.

There are many forms of periodisation. Some people simply vary the intensity of their lifting over a weekly period:

Workout 1—heavy (3-5RM)
Workout 2—light (12-15RM)
Workout 3—medium (8-10RM)

Another way for highly motivated trainers is to work at 100% intensity for the three workouts but change the exercise to fit the heavy-light-medium paradigm. For example, a trainer may select three exercises that overload the shoulder girdle (bench press, military press and incline press) and vary the weight to suit the exercise.

The underlying concept of periodisation is the use of training cycles. This means that the trainer should start with high volume, low intensity work. This is followed with low volume work while increasing intensity to maximum. This technique attempts to maximise strength/power while minimising the probability of over training.

A popular periodisation model, adapted from the work of Stone, O'Bryant and Garhammer, follows a linear intensification approach to strength development (Table 6.4).

Table 6.4: A Model for Strength Training

Preparation	Transition 1	Competition	Transition 2	
		Basic	Strength	Peaking* or
Phase	Hypertrophy	strength	and power	maintenance
Sets†	3–5	3–5	3–5	1–3
Reps	8–20	2–6	2–3	1–3
Days/week	3–4	3–5	4–6	1–5
Time/day	1–3	1–3	1–2	1
Intensity cycle (weeks)**	2–3/1	2–4/1	2–3/1	—
Intensity	low	high	high to low	very high
Volume	high	moderate to high	low	very low

*   Peaking for sports with a definite climax or maintenance for sports with a long season such as football.

**   Ratio of the number of heavy training weeks to light training weeks.

†   Does not include warm-up sets.

Another approach to periodisation is alternating moderate weeks before more intense weeks in two weekly training blocks.

Weeks	1–2	3–4	5–6	7–8	9–10	11–12
Reps	10–12	4–6	8–10	3–5	6–8	2–3
Sets	3	5	4	5	4	6
Intensity*	70–75% (1RM)	82–88%	75–78%	85–90%	80–85%	90–95%
Volume**	30–36	20–30	32–40	15–25	24–32	12–18

*   Intensity refers to the percentage of the 1RM being lifted in a workout.

**   Volume can be defined as the total number of repetitions performed in a workout or the total amount of weight lifted in a workout (sets × reps × load).

Frequency of Workout

The amount of recovery between workouts should be dependent on the recovery ability of the individual. Traditionally three workouts per week (Mon–Wed–Fri) is considered to be optimal.

The Split Routine

With more experienced lifters it is not practical to use the traditional three workouts per week schedule as the training sessions would be far too long. The split routine overcomes this problem by dividing the training session into body parts. The most common form is the four day per week split, also called the 'push and pull' workout. This is as follows:

• Pushing movements are done on Mondays and Thursdays, emphasising chest, shoulders and triceps.
• Pulling movements are done on Tuesdays and Fridays, emphasising legs, back and triceps.

There are many other variations of the split routine, but with most there is a definite risk of over training due to the amount and intensity of work that can be done in each training session.

Classification and Choice of Exercise

1. Isolation exercises These usually isolate a single specific muscle across one joint. For example, dumbell lateral raise, pec flyes and concentration curl.

2. Compound exercises These exercises involve the use of many muscles and joints to produce movement. For example, bench press, squat and power clean.

Table 6.5: Selection of Exercises

Major muscles	Compound	Isolation	Major muscles	Compound	Isolation
Pectoralis major	Bench press Incline press	DB flyes Cable work	Gluteus maximus	Lunge	Total hip
			Spinae erector	Deadlift Good morning	Hyperextension
Latissimus dorsi	Bent over row Lat pulldown	DB pullover	Gastrocnemius Soleus	Skipping	Calf raises
Deltoids	Press behind neck Upright row	DB raises 3 sides: 1. anterior 2. lateral 3. posterior	Bicep brachii	Close grip chins Bar curls	Preacher curls Concentration Curls
			Triceps brachii	Close grip bench press Dips	Pressdowns Kickbacks
Quadriceps	Squats	Leg extension			
Hamstrings	Dead lift	Leg curl			

Safety Precautions in Resistance Training

1. When lifting weights from the floor, bench or table:

• Stand with the feet parallel, shoulder width apart and close to the bar
• Lower the hips by flexing the knees
• Maintain a straight back, held as vertical as possible
• Keep the head up
• Lift the weight by extending or straightening the legs.

2. Before beginning each exercise, be sure the feet are properly positioned, the pelvis is stabilised and the hands gripping the bar are an equal distance apart from each end of the bar.

3. Always wipe the benches down after use and return the weights to their racks. Always dismantle weights after use e.g. the squat bar or the bench press bar.

4. Watch for frayed cables or loose collars on bars.

5. When lifting weights participants should:

• Be familiar with the equipment they wish to use
• Use the correct lifting techniques
• Know their limits
• Never drop the weights after use
• Grip the weight correctly prior to the lift
• Load and unload the equipment correctly.

Choosing the Best Equipment

When weight training, there is a variety of machines and training systems available. While the manufacturers of each often claim special advantages, no one machine system caters for all contingencies. All have their advantages and disadvantages and there is even controversy over the use of free weights versus machines.

For Free Weights

1. Transfer of training Specificity of training is a key aspect of strength and fitness development for sports. With free weights, it has been suggested that the individual's own pattern of motor unit firing, used in non weight training performance, can be stimulated closely through isotonic movements. This is because the freely moving bar is not being 'guided' or otherwise restrained as would be the case with machine movement and because the resistance throughout the range of movement is similar to that in normal activities and not artificially isokinetic. Training would then be expected to better transfer to 'the real world'.

2. Joint strength Because the free weight user has to balance the resistance rather than be guided by machinery, the controlling action may be an aid in developing joint strength. Says University of Hawaii strength coach Bill Starr: 'As a football player takes a loaded barbell off the bench press stand, he must steady the bar before lowering it to the chest. The controlling action builds tendon and ligament strength in the wrist, elbow and shoulder joints.'

3. Muscle synergism In normal movements, a number of 'synergist' or supporting muscles aid the prime mover. Many exercise machines, however, are constructed to isolate one or a limited number of muscles and work intensively on these. Free weights, it is argued, offer better total muscle group conditioning than machine systems, therefore offering greater economy of training.

4. Individuality Some machines are designed to provide variable resistance through the full range of movement. However, to do so, they rely on force–angle relationships which are based on estimates from the average person. Individual differences in limb strength, point of muscle attachment, muscle architecture, velocity of movement etc. mean that certain individuals may be restricted in their movements because inappropriate workloads may be applied at various angles. This does not occur with free weights.

5. Psychological factors Although not proven, it has been suggested that athletes are more motivated to improve their strength performance on free weights. This is because of the greater satisfaction of improving

poundage and personal best performances with loose weights.

For the Machine Systems

1. Safety Because machine systems are generally attached within a unit there are safety advantages that are not present with heavy loose weights. This is particularly so with non-weight hydraulic systems where children may be present. Some manufacturers also claim that there is less chance of injury through incorrect movements if the range of movements is fixed.

2. Cheating As for safety, the fixed movements of many weight systems ensure that an exercise is carried out correctly and that cheating cannot occur. This is a particular advantage for beginners and those who tend to take the easy way out.

3. Compactness There's little question that most machine systems are more compact and neat, and therefore more physically attractive in many gym situations than loose weights. They also offer the advantage that many people can be trained simultaneously. However, the latter claim needs to be seen in perspective, because cost differentials mean that many barbells and dumbells could be purchased for the price of one multi-station unit.

4. Rehabilitation training The guided action and variable resistance of some machine systems makes them particularly suited to injury rehabilitation training. Less strain is likely to be put on injured joints than with free weights.

5. General fitness training Where specific muscle strength, as in sport training, is not the aim of the program, machine systems maybe of more advantage than free weights. Certain systems may be of particular advantage in circuit training.

Resistance Training and Women

Women do not have the same capabilities to increase muscular size as men due to the fact that the average female has ten times less testosterone in her system than the average male. This is paralleled by the fact that female muscle produces less tension per unit volume and has a smaller cross sectional area in each muscle fibre.

Women have the same potential for strength

development as men although it is through a different mechanism. Females increase their strength by improving the recruitment of motor nerves rather than altering the contractile structures of their muscles.

Some research has shown that when males and females are compared using the method of strength per unit of lean body mass, females are in fact slightly stronger than men in certain areas such as the hips and

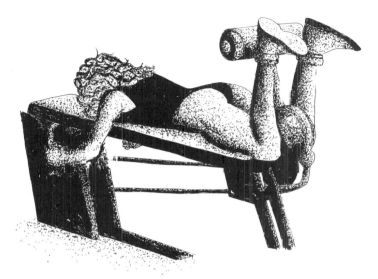

legs. However, until recently, women have shied away from weight training because of their fear of developing large bulging muscles. There is now considerable research that has allayed many of these concerns.

Women can weight train without fear of muscle hypertrophy.

In a study carried out by Dr Jack Wilmore in 1974, a group of untrained college men and women were given a 10 week weight training program. Before training, the women's strength was around 25-28% lower than that of the man, although when body weight was taken into consideration, there were no sex differences in strength. After training, strength improved significantly (i.e. 5-25%) and equally in both groups. Yet while muscle size increased significantly in the men, there was no significant increase in size for women.

Muscle tone and body shape on the other hand may be significantly enhanced by weight training in women because of changes that can occur in fat/muscle ratio. Research on muscle size difference with training between men and women is shown in Figure. 6.11.

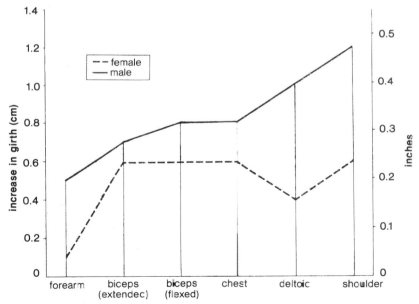

Fig. 6.11: Muscular hypertrophy in females is generally not as great as in males even when the same strength gains have been made. (From Fox 1979).

Prepubescent Strength Training

The National Strength and Conditioning Association's (NSCA) position paper on prepubescent strength training has prepared guidelines which state that strength training may begin at any age. It states that commencement age is dependent on the child undergoing a physical examination and on him having the emotional maturity to take direction from the trainer. Further research is required, but at present the use of higher repetitions and sets with lower loads is most appropriate. The NSCA recommends 6–15 repetitions per set and 1RM testing should never be attempted at this age.

A model training session for prepubescent children should be performed 3 times per week. Each session should consist of a warm up, 30 min weight exercises, 20 min run, 20 min team game, then a cool down. The session should stress total body development and should include exercises using the child's own body-weight such as dips and chins.

Further requirements on weight training for adolescents have been listed in a position paper by the Australian Sports Medicine Federation in 1989.

Variations in Weight Training from the Beginner to the Advanced

Techniques and prescription are two vital aspects of any weight-training program. Most standard instructional weight training texts have set approaches to both.

Yet just as a beginner would not be given the same amount of weight to lift as an advanced exerciser, there are lifting techniques which also change with experience. Some of these are not covered in the standard texts. For example:

1. Feet positioning in the bench press: Commercially made bench-press benches are often long enough only to accommodate the torso to the base of the pelvis in the supine position.

This means the legs are left to hang over the edge of the bench. The legs can either be positioned flat on the floor, in which case the back is arched, or placed in the air or on the end of the bench, thus flattening the back.

An arched (and unsupported) back is potentially dangerous for the inexperienced or those with lower back problems. Hence, the beginner should be taught either to raise the feet to an extension of the bench, or cross the legs in the air so the back is flattened (Figure 6.12). On the other hand, an experienced lifter using a heavy weight may need to keep the feet flat on the floor for extra support.

2. Use of machines versus free weights: Machine systems in resistance training have a distinct safety advantage over free weights. Because the action is guided, it is more difficult for the beginner to carry out an exercise incorrectly. It is also more appropriate for learning the correct technique for later progression to free weights.

Free weights offer advantages over machine systems in that support muscles are used, joints are strengthened and the action is more like 'real life'.

The correct progression then would be from machine systems to free weights where the actions are duplicated.

3. Progressions in the squat: The squat is one of the best overall compound exercises available. But it has inherent dangers, particularly because of the pressure placed on knee ligaments when the knee is flexed beyond 90 degrees. Orthopaedic studies have shown that the shearing force on the knee can increase by up to 7 times that of the weight being carried when the knee is flexed beyond this position.

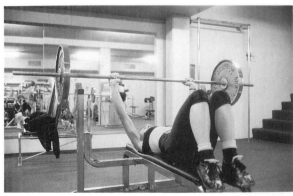

Fig. 6.12: Raise the legs for the bench press to ensure a flat back

Other problems with the squat are:

• The difficulty in performing the exact technique such that the maximum benefits are gained
• The tendency to cheat in order to carry a heavy load.

For the beginner, any of the standard squat machines can help develop technique. However, the beginner should never be put into the full squat position.

Often, lack of flexibility in the Achilles tendon leads to a tendency to want to place the heels on a raised block. But this only exacerbates the problem. The beginner then should be taught to squat only to a point that is comfortable with the heels on the floor and not beyond the position of thighs parallel to the floor. As flexibility improves, allowing greater movement, the squat can, with caution, be taken lower.

Other changes which can be made with advanced training include changes in feet position (toes in/out etc.), changes in the position of the bar (back of neck versus front of chest), and changes in weight used.

4. Increased sets/decreased reps: In the early part of a weight-training program, large increases in strength can come from one set of relatively low-resistance exercises. This has the added advantage of minimising muscle soreness and reducing the risk of injury.

Only with experience should the weight be increased while ensuring correct technique. Repetitions can be decreased from 15–20 per set to 6–8 per set and weight increased accordingly. Sets can then be increased to provide muscle overload once muscle groups have adapted.

5. From uniformity to periodisation: For a beginner, the most important aspect of a weight-training program is learning technique and muscle adaptation. Hence, uniformity of a training program over 3–4 days a week is important, with gradual progressions in resistance, repetitions etc.

For the more advanced exerciser on the other hand, greater advances are made from periodisation; that is changing the program over a set period of either weeks or months.

A regime of light weights with high repetitions can be used for 3–6 weeks, followed by a period of 3–6 weeks with heavy weights and low repetitions. This can then lead into a third cycle, where the weight is relatively light again, although at a higher level than phase 1. Greater strength developments have been shown using this technique than the uniform training approach.

6. From 'compound' to 'isolation': Isolation exercises (i.e. those using predominantly a prime mover muscle) have little value to a beginning exerciser looking for increases in aerobic fitness as well as general improvements in muscle tone.

Energy usage in isolation work is generally lower than with compound exercises (i.e. those with more than one muscle or group involved). With improved general fitness more isolation work may be included in order to improve on specific muscle development. Hence the beginner would concentrate on compound movements, the advanced on a compound/isolation mix.

7. Learn lifting technique before progressing to heavy weight: Ensure the lifter has mastered the techique with lighter weights so that he/she can progress to heavier weights with good form. This will prevent additional muscles being recruited when lifting heavier weights. Take for example the squat where an inexperienced lifter using too heavy a weight will have the tendency to forward flex the trunk, while at the same time losing some stability at the knee joints causing them to come together.

8. For the beginner: Stress caution and avoid exercises involving hyperextension and extreme joint flexion.

9. Breathe normally throughout the lift: As a general rule, lifters should exhale with the exertion and inhale when lowering the weight. However, there are exceptions to this rule. Take for example an upright row where it does not feel right to breathe out when lifting the weight to the chin and to breathe in when lowering the weight. To overcome these exceptions instructors should encourage participants to keep their mouths open, and to breathe normally throughout the lift.

If a weight trainer does not breathe correctly during a lift, blood pressure can increase dramatically due to what is called a 'valsalva' manoeuvre. This means making an expiratory effort with the glottis closed (the glottis is the space or opening between the vocal cords). Since air cannot escape, intrathoracic pressure increases appreciably, even to the point where it can cause the venae cavae, which returns blood to the heart, to collapse. This in turn can cause the person to black out.

Guidelines for Weight Training

The following are some guidelines for the administration of weight training programs:

1. At least 5 minutes of warm-up (see Chapter 4) should be carried out before lifting weights. This includes stretching and loosening up exercises of gradually increasing intensity.

2. Particular attention should be paid to safety and to correct exercise procedure. Individual counselling is advisable to assess structural weakness or abnormalities in participants.

3. Weight standards should be determined at the outset for each participant. These should then be adjusted according to improvement.

4. A strength training routine should involve the use of the overload principle, i.e. progressively heavier weights or an increasing number of repetitions and/or sets.

5. Strength training should not be confused with aerobic conditioning and no suggestion should be made that strength training or body building alone will significantly improve aerobic fitness.

6. Heavy resistances should not be used until proper lifting techniques are perfected.

7. Individual record cards should be available for participants so that workouts can be standardised and efforts recorded. Regular monitoring of cards by an instructor and regular consultations with the client should be carried out.

8. Opposing (agonist/antagonist) muscle groups should be involved in all exercises to ensure balanced development.

9. Caution should be used in relation to back hyperextension exercises, and doing full squats with heavy resistances.

10. The pelvis should be stabilised on all exercises and the body should be positioned correctly before starting each exercise.

11. Each exercise should be performed with a smooth, even rhythm, moving the weight(s) through the full range of joint movement.

12. Correct breathing is important. Inhalation should occur on the lifting of the weight and exhalation on lowering. The breath should not be held at any time.

13. Make training as interesting as possible to avoid boredom and maintain motivation in training.

14. Exercise large muscle groups before smaller ones.

15. Allow adequate recovery between individual exercises and workouts to ensure the muscles are well rested for the next workout.

16. At least 3 or 4 workouts per week should be performed to improve fitness.

17. If in doubt about the proper technique of an exercise seek instruction; do not resort to trial and error.

7 Mechanics of Movement and Potentially Dangerous Exercises

The fitness boom has seen a big increase in over-use or chronic injuries due to exercise, which were virtually unheard of a decade ago. It is essential therefore that anyone involved in exercise programming has an understanding of why some exercises are considered to be potentially dangerous and what alternatives can be used.

In this chapter we'll examine some basic mechanics of the musculo-skeletal system in order to clarify why some exercises are considered to be 'better' than others, and more specifically, which exercises might be potentially harmful.

The Dangers of Exercise

In any architectural or mechanical structure, certain components are continuously placed under stress or strain. If this becomes too great through over-use or simply with age, weaknesses are likely to develop. An analogy is in driving a motor car: if a car is only driven on short trips at a moderate pace, minor structural weaknesses can be masked. But if it is taken on a long drive at speed, any minor defects are likely to show up.

So it is with the body. At mild exercise levels, small structural defects such as differences in leg length (which are surprisingly common), are unlikely to be noticed. But if the exerciser then takes up endurance exercise for example, chronic injury is likely to result.

Even for the structurally sound, some exercises can place excessive strain on muscles and joints. If this happens, wear and tear can result, degenerative changes may set in and damage may be irreparable.

The Mechanics of Joint and Muscle Action

To enable the body to improve its mechanical efficiency during movement, skeletal muscles employ simple mechanical principles such as the lever system. All lever systems have a fulcrum (the joint), a rigid lever arm (the bone) and require force through a muscular contraction.

The position of the joint (the fulcrum) in relation to the muscles determines the type of lever system being used.

There are three main types of levers in the body:

1. First Class Lever
The fulcrum (joint) always lies between the effort (muscle) and the resistance (weight). This is the most

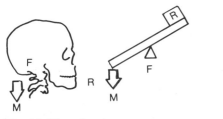

Fig. 7.1: First class lever

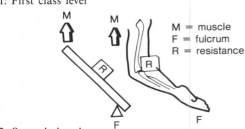

M = muscle
F = fulcrum
R = resistance

Fig. 7.2: Second class lever

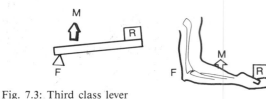

Fig. 7.3: Third class lever

efficient form of lever (Figure 7.1), an example being the movement of the head.

2. Second Class Lever

In this instance the resistance (R) always lies between the fulcrum (F) and the effort (M) (Figure 7.2). An example would be pushing or lifting a wheelbarrow or lifting the body weight up onto the toes.

3. Third Class Lever

Here the muscular effort is placed between the weight and the joint, providing the least efficient mechanical advantage (Figure 7.3). An example is the contraction of the biceps to lift the hand.

If excessive strain (force or weight) is applied to the lever in any of these three systems, the force placed on the fulcrum is increased, resulting in wear and tear on the joint. Hence the aim of an exercise program should be to maximise the strength and efficiency of the muscles while minimising the detrimental forces to the fulcrum (or joint).

Importance of a Balanced Exercise Program

Skeletal muscles have different functions depending on their location in the body. The muscles that support the body when standing, sitting or lying are called 'postural' muscles and are active for long periods of time. The muscles that generate and maintain movement are called 'phasic' muscles and work in association with the postural muscles.

Examples of phasic and postural muscles of the lower trunk and legs are:

Postural muscles	Phasic muscles
Erector spinae group	Rectus abdominus
Tibialis posterior	Obliques
Tensor fasciae latae	Gluteus maximus
Iliopsoas	Vastus medialis
Rectus femoris	Gluteus medius and minimus
Piriformis	Tibialis anterior
Adductors	Peroneus brevis and longus
Hamstring group	
Gastrocnemius and soleus	
Quadratus lumborum	

When designing exercise programs an understanding of the function of postural and phasic muscles is important for the following reasons:

1. Postural muscles are stronger than phasic. So, before phasic muscles can be exercised, postural muscles must be relaxed.

2. Sedentary living can cause an imbalance between postural and phasic. Someone who is 'deskbound' all day may have strong back extensor muscles (postural) and weak abdominal muscles (phasic). This can make that person predisposed to lower back pain.

3. With increasing age, the postural muscles tighten while the phasic muscles weaken. When designing programs for older people therefore, postural should be stretched and phasic strengthened.

Potentially Dangerous Exercises

Aerobics and fitness training is a rapidly changing field. Only in the last five to ten years have exercise scientists looked closely at the benefits and concerns of relatively new exercise forms such as exercise to music classes. As the fitness industry continues to grow and more unfit, overweight, sedentary individuals take up aerobics, the experts are finding it necessary to identify which exercises tend to cause injury. To make sure that classes are effective and safe, fitness instructors *must* be up-to-date not only on potentially dangerous exercises, but *why* the danger exists and *how* to modify the exercises.

Understand

Consistency in an industry adds credibility. If all fitness instructors have a sound understanding of what constitutes an exercise danger, programs will become safer and participants will not be asking 'why does one instructor often do that exercise and now I am told it's dangerous?'

The first step to providing safer exercise programs is a *willingness to change*. Just because an instructor has been doing an exercise for a long time doesn't mean the exercise is safe. Instructors should keep in mind that there are *no lists* which contain every potentially dangerous exercise. Instructors must try to *understand* the elements which increase risk and the areas where injuries are most likely to occur. Then, each instructor can evaluate their own exercises and determine which ones need to be modified.

There are conflicting opinions, even among 'the experts' about which exercises are dangerous. If an instructor has a clear understanding of *why* a movement may be dangerous, he/she can then listen to conflicting opinions and make an educated decision.

Fitness instructors should keep in mind three primary factors:

The participants Every individual is different in terms of strength, flexibility, skill, coordination, weight, fitness level and speed of learning. Some may be more prone to injury because of anatomical, structural or other physiological factors. Often these factors may be present without the individual (and hence the instructor) being aware of them. Exercise safety is a priority in all programs. A very fit person can be just as injury prone as an unfit one.

Also, wearing the wrong shoes or no shoes at all

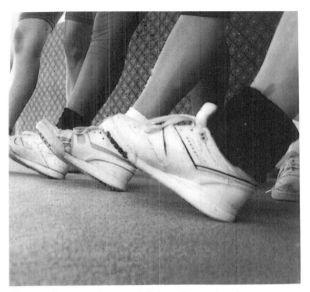

Correct footwear is essential for all exercise classes

is a potential danger, and a leading cause of lower leg pain and injury. Try to avoid letting people exercise bare-footed, and encourage the wearing of proper, well designed shoes. There is no such thing as the perfect shoe that is suitable for everyone.

The instructor The instructor can control the degree of safety of an exercise. Speed of movement, number of repetitions, sequencing of exercises, cueing of changes, and amount of impact are all controllable. The instructor who is up-to-date understands these variables and uses them effectively when planning programs.

The goal The primary goal of the exercise program is to improve physical fitness as well as improving some psychological aspects such as self-esteem, and sense of accomplishment. Leaving an exercise program with a sore back, sore knees, uncomfortable shins, or feeling overly exhausted does not encourage anyone to return. For fitness instructors to encourage *life long* fitness, programs have to be safe, effective, and painless. Remember that there is a difference between *pain* and *overload*. Cardiovascular or muscular overload is necessary to improve the level of fitness, and while this may be accompanied by a slight discomfort, it should not be painful. In fact a good rule of thumb is: *If it hurts, don't do it!*

Evaluate

The elements which tend to cause injury are:

Extreme movements Movements which go beyond a safe range of motion either in distance or direction. Most movements which involve hyperflexion and hyperextension are considered extreme. For example, the 'cobra stretch' (lying face down, hands under the shoulders and fully extending the arms, pushing up to bend the back) places the lower back in an extreme extended position (Figure 7.4). The use of momentum during exercise may also lead to extreme ranges of motion at the moving joint—this is referred to as ballistic movement.

Ballistic movements Movements performed rapidly, without control, going beyond the normal range of motion. Often an exercise may be safe, but when performed rapidly, becomes unsafe. For example, rapidly swinging the arms to mobilise the shoulders (Figure 7.5). This places stress on the connective tissue in the shoulder joint and does not promote mobility or flexibility.

Excessive load Movements may involve excessive load to a joint or muscle group. For example, 'power jumps'—jumping up and touching the floor with the hands. On landing, an excessive load is applied to the knees if they are forced to bend beyond a safe (90 degree) angle (Figure 7.6 (a) & (b)).

Sustained movements Any movement or position that involves a sustained stress on a muscle group of joint. For example, sitting in a V-sit position with feet on the floor and the back unsupported (free back) to work the abdominal muscles (Figure 7.7). In this position, there is excessive, sustained load on the lower back from the heavy upper body lever, causing high intervertebral pressure. The result: lower back pain.

Repetitive movements Excessive repetitions (even of safe exercises) can cause pain, discomfort and injury. During floorwork, change exercises frequently before pain is felt in any one muscle group. During aerobic work, use no more than 32 consecutive footstrike patterns and no more than 8 consecutive footstrikes on one leg (as in 4 consecutive knee lifts on one leg) (Figure 7.8).

Imbalance Working one muscle group excessively without working the opposing muscle group, or, exercises in which the primary mover is stronger than the muscle which you are trying to work. For example, the iliopsoas muscle (hip flexor) is six to eight times stronger than the rectus abdominis. As such, the bicycling motion (Figure 7.9) which is often thought

to strengthen the lower abdominals is generated mainly by the hip flexors.

A second example is the lack of tibialis anterior strengthening and stretching to balance the calf work often done in aerobic classes. This can cause a muscular imbalance which may lead to pain in the lower leg.

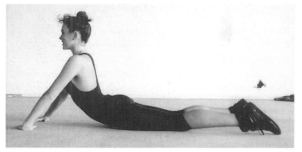
Fig. 7.4: Cobra Stretch—extreme hyperextension

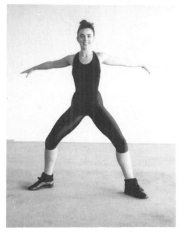
Fig. 7.5: Only use controlled movements when moving rapidly

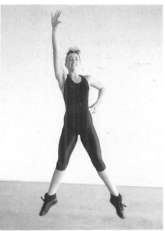
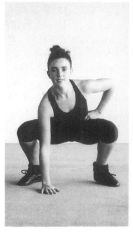
Fig. 7.6: a) Power jump b) On landing excessive load can be placed on the knees

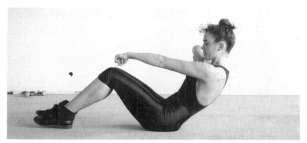

Fig. 7.7: V sits or free back are not recommended

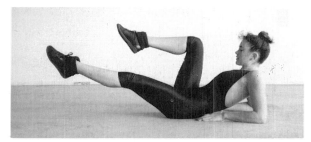

Fig. 7.9: Bicycling—a hip flexor exercise more than an abdominal exercise

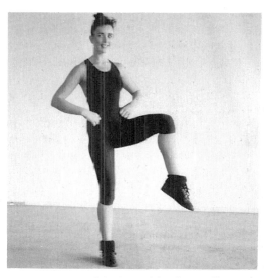

Fig. 7.8: Be careful of repetitive foot strike movements

Principles of Movement

In addition to these elements that increase risk, there are several principles of movement (and physics!) which must be understood:

The force of gravity Gravity can be used to advantage in some exercises but in others it can increase risk. Because of gravity, the force applied to a joint can be increased. For example, standing in a forward flexed position to stretch the hamstrings causes a substantial rise in disc pressure and increases the strain on back extensor muscles and ligaments. A much safer hamstring stretch can be achieved in a lying position (Figure 7.10). Movements that involve jumping (which should be done in moderation and combined with non-jumping movements) also increase joint stress, as do positions that involve long, heavy, or inefficient lever systems, such as free back and double leg raises.

Gravity can work in our favour by providing a small amount of 'built in resistance'. For example, abdominal crunches involve lifting the upper body against the force of gravity, hence increasing the effectiveness of the exercise.

Joint stresses Our whole body functions as a system of levers. Long levers (i.e., straight legs and arms) require more muscular involvement than short levers (i.e., bent legs and arms) hence placing additional stresses on the joints. For example, 'Rover's revenge' with a straight leg out to the side is a long lever

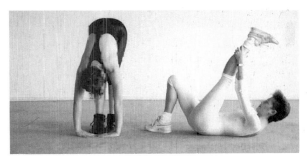

Fig. 7.10: Toe touching to stretch the hamstrings—a safer alternative is in the lying position

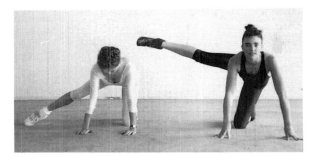

Fig. 7.11: Rover's Revenge—long lever and the safer short lever alternative

movement placing stress on the lower back. This exercise becomes safer when the leg does not have to move through such a large range of motion i.e., starting with a bent knee and touching the toe to the floor only (Figure 7.11). Figures 7.12 and 7.13 show additional long lever positions which place high stress on the lower back. Combining short and long lever movements and shortening the lever when joint stress is suspected will make your work-outs safer.

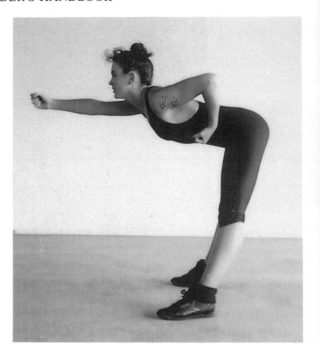

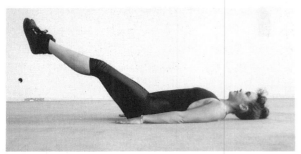

Fig. 7.12 and 7.13: Long lever exercises that place stress on the lower back

The Final Step in Evaluation

Each of the elements and the movement mechanics above are related to the *risk* of an exercise. The final step in the evaluation process is to consider the effectiveness of the movement. Ask yourself why you are doing the exercise—aerobic conditioning, muscular strength, endurance, flexibility, mobility? Then determine what muscle group you are trying to work. Does the exercise accomplish these things? There are several possible relationships between risk and effectiveness:

Low effectiveness/low risk These are typically the 'filler' exercises in your work-out. For example, lying on your back and kicking the legs up in the air like a 'dead bug' (Figure 7.14). These exercises are not necessarily dangerous, but they don't have a real purpose either. Try to replace them with exercises that work specific muscle groups and provide an overload in a short period of time.

Low effectiveness/high risk Rolling the neck backwards (Figure 7.15) has no real benefit (the front of the neck is not an area that commonly needs to be stretched) and has a very high risk (stress on the cervical vertebrae). Exercises that fall into this category definitely need to be replaced!

High effectiveness/high risk These exercises are effective, but the risk associated with them makes them

potentially dangerous. An example is the sprint start position (Figure 7.16) when used for cardiovascular conditioning. Heart rate can definitely reach a training zone, but there are several risks associated with this position. Regardless of the fitness level of your participants, modify or remove these exercises from the program.

High effectiveness/low risk The ideal combination! All exercises in your program should fall into this category. Aerobic exercises should be strenuous enough for people to achieve their target heart rates, but not so strenuous that they are working at a fatigue level, susceptible to injury or discomfort. Floor exercises should be done in a slow, controlled manner, working full range of motion, providing overload within a short period of time, and with limited repetitions and frequent changes of position.

Modify

The final step in providing safe and effective classes is to *modify* the potentially dangerous exercises.

The feeling of frustration is high when you first discover that half the exercises you've been doing for years are dangerous. Remember that for every exercise you take out of your classes to increase safety, there is an alternative exercise. It may mean modifying a position, or changing a position altogether, but there

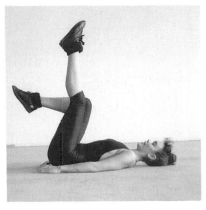

Fig. 7.14: Dead Bug—not dangerous but ineffective

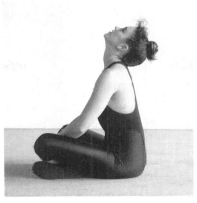

Fig. 7.15: Neck hyperextension places excessive stress on the cervical vertebrae

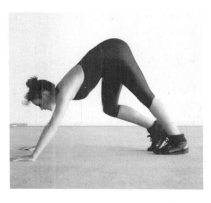

Fig. 7.16: Sprint Start—problems with dizziness, blood pressure and shoulders

is always an alternative. Go back to the question you asked yourself, 'Why am I doing this exercise?' If it was for abdominal toning, what are some other ways you can achieve that goal with less risk? Sometimes making the program (e.g. an aerobic class) safer is simply a matter of slowing down the pace! Slower, controlled movements working full range of motion will always be safer and more effective than rapid ones in both aerobic and floor work. Besides, what's the hurry? A good aerobic exercise class should be a work-out not a wipe-out!

Use the following 'Safer Moves' segment as a guideline for areas in which potentially dangerous exercises occur. Remember, there are so many exercises, variations and combinations that no list will ever include all the dangerous exercises. It is up to the instructor to understand, evaluate and modify!

Safer Moves

Key The model in black is doing the dangerous exercise, the model in white a modified safe version.

Head and Neck

Momentum
Avoid rapid or jerking movements (Figure 7.17). Instead, use controlled movement from side to side or up and down.

Hyperextension
Neck rolls or stretches in the back direction should be avoided due to stress on the cervical vertebrae (Figure 7.18). When doing exercises on all fours there is a tendency to hyperextend the neck to see the instructor (Figure 7.19). Turn side-on, maintain a neutral head position rotating it slightly to observe the instructor. Also avoid hyperextension during abdominal work (Figure 7.20).

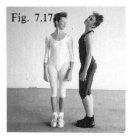

Fig. 7.17

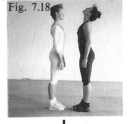

Fig. 7.18

Fig. 7.19

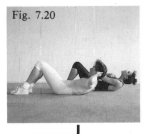

Fig. 7.20

Momentum   **Hyperextension**

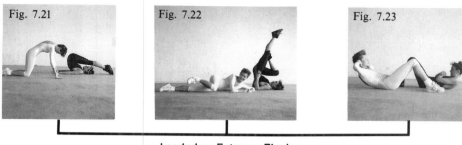

Loaded or Extreme Flexion

Loaded or extreme flexion

This also causes excessive stress on the cervical vertebrae. Replace the 'plough' with the cat stretch (Figure 7.21). Avoid standing on the shoulders at all times (Figure 7.22). Encourage participants not to pull the head when supporting it during abdominal work (Figure 7.23). Avoid pulling the head to stretch the back of the neck.

Shoulders

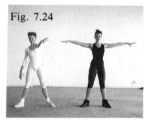

Sustained Repetitive
Isolations

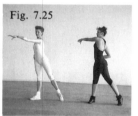

Momentum

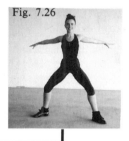

Impingements

Sustained, repetitive shoulder isolations

Small movements with the arms out to the side are examples of repeated shoulder isolations (Figure 7.24). Work full range of motion, varying between short and long levers.

Momentum

Rapidly swinging the shoulders places undue stress on the shoulder joint without much benefit (Figure 7.25a and 7.26). Work within the normal range of motion and try to avoid any rapid swinging or pulling movements.

Impingement

Excessive, repetitive (normally more than fifty) arm movements in the same direction, particularly overhead (Figure 7.27) or to the front or side can cause impingement in the shoulder area. Limit the number of repetitions and change arm positions frequently. In addition, keep the arms slightly forward rather than straight overhead in upward movements.

Trunk/Torso

Free back

Supporting the heavy upper body in this position (Figure 7.28) causes high intervertebral pressure and stress on the lower back. In addition, to effectively work the abdominals, they should generally be worked through a full range of motion, rather than sustaining an isometric contraction. The danger is increased further when a twisting motion is added (Figure 7.29) or when the feet are off the ground as in the 'jackknife' position (Figure 7.30).

Double straight leg raises

Supporting the long lever of the legs in this position (Figure 7.31) causes stress on the lower back and can lead to back pain. Also avoid variations of this position such as scissors and flutter kicks (Figure 7.32). Because the prime mover is the hip flexors the abdominals receive little benefit from these exercises.

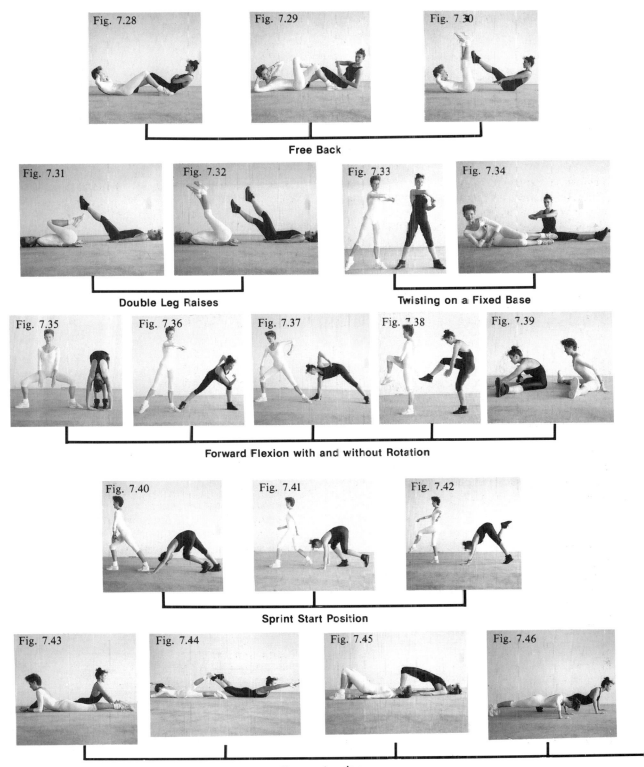

Fig. 7.28 Fig. 7.29 Fig. 7.30

Free Back

Fig. 7.31 Fig. 7.32

Double Leg Raises

Fig. 7.33 Fig. 7.34

Twisting on a Fixed Base

Fig. 7.35 Fig. 7.36 Fig. 7.37 Fig. 7.38 Fig. 7.39

Forward Flexion with and without Rotation

Fig. 7.40 Fig. 7.41 Fig. 7.42

Sprint Start Position

Fig. 7.43 Fig. 7.44 Fig. 7.45 Fig. 7.46

Hyperextension

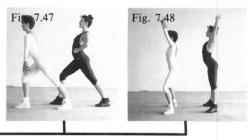

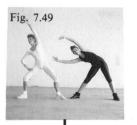

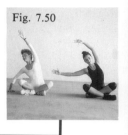

Hyperextension cont'd

Excessive Lateral Flexion

Twisting on a fixed base

These movements apply excessive rotational torque to the lower back. When standing and twisting (Figure 7.33), one heel should be raised. Rapid and/or repetitive twisting should not be performed when seated (Figure 7.34). It is more effective to perform slow, controlled twisting movements with the back safely supported on the floor.

Forward flexion with and without rotation

Forward flexion (Figure 7.35) increases pressure on the discs and ligaments of the lower back by more than three times body weight. Rotation with forward flexion (Figure 7.36) further increases torque and pressure. Tricep and rhomboid exercises should be done more upright (Figure 7.37). Clapping under the thigh can encourage forward flexion (Figure 7.38) so a straight back position should be encouraged, or modify the exercise by clapping on top of the thigh. When seated to stretch the adductor or hamstring muscles (Figure 7.39), the back should remain straight, not rounded. If stretching the back, controlled rounding should be done with knees bent or crossed.

Sprint start position

Commonly used to stretch the calves and for aerobic work. This position has at least three potential dangers: the neck is hyperextended to see the instructor; or, if

lowered, falls below the level of the heart causing a blood rush to the head; and there is a sustained isometric contraction of the arms to support the body causing both discomfort and increased chest pressure which can result in cardiovascular irregularities. Stretch the calves in a seated or standing position (Figure 7.40) and do the aerobic work upright (Figures 7.41 and 7.42)—it is just as effective!

Hyperextension

While some back hyperextension work is necessary to strengthen its muscles and stretch the opposing muscle groups, pain can result if the position is extreme. When extending the back in a prone position go no further than resting on the elbows (Figure 7.43). Avoid lifting both upper and lower body off the ground simultaneously, alternate instead (Figure 7.44). Keep the back on the ground during pelvic tilts (Figure 7.45). Avoid sagging the abdominal area when doing on-all-fours leg work or pushups (Figure 7.46). Be careful not to hyperextend in exercises such as calf stretches or shoulder work (Figures 7.47 and 7.48).

Excessive lateral flexion

Bending too far to the side without support (standing or seated— Figures 7.49 and 7.50) places stress on the lower back from a lateral angle. Always use the arm for support.

Hip

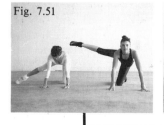

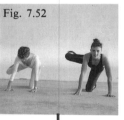

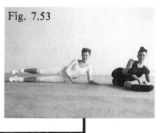

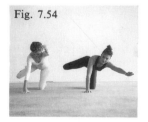

Abduction at 90° angle

Balance Test

Abduction at 90 degree angle

Holding and moving a straight leg out to the side when on all fours places high stresses on the lower back (Figure 7.51). Even with a bent knee, the rotational stress on the lower back is high if the movement is extreme (Figure 7.52). To reduce stress, limit the range of motion to within the balance test (see below) When lying on the side in an L-shaped position, stress to the back and hip area is also high (Figure 7.53). Bend at the hips no more than 45 degrees.

Balance test

To be sure your hip work is safe, use the balance test (Figure 7.54). Never move the leg higher than the point at which you are evenly balanced when the opposite arm is raised to the front.

Knee

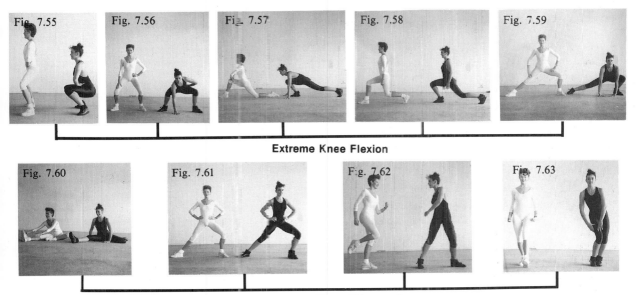

Fig. 7.55   Fig. 7.56   Fig. 7.57   Fig. 7.58   Fig. 7.59

Extreme Knee Flexion

Fig. 7.60   Fig. 7.61   Fig. 7.62   Fig. 7.63

Incorrect Knee Alignment

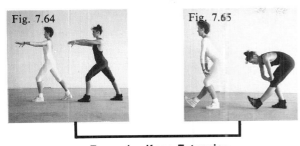

Fig. 7.64   Fig. 7.65

Excessive Knee Extension

Deep knee bends and other positions of extreme knee flexion

High stresses are placed on the knee joint if it is bent beyond 90 degrees. Deep squats (Figure 7.55), power jumps where the end position is touching the floor (Figure 7.56), hip flexor stretches with hands on the floor (Figure 7.57), stepping into a lunge (Figure 7.58), adductor stretching where the knee is excessively bent (Figure 7.59), and burpees, can all cause potential damage.

Incorrect knee alignment

The hurdler's stretch (Figure 7.60), poor technique in side to side movement (Figure 7.61), rapid directional changes (Figure 7.62) and knee circling (Figure 7.63) may all cause a twisting of the knee which can lead to injury. Slow down directional changes, align the centre of the knee directly over the middle of the foot when bending and make sure rotation comes from the hip, not the knee.

Excessive knee extension

Locking the knee when stepping behind in L.I.A. movements (Figure 7.64) and leaning on the knee of a straight leg (Figure 7.65) can cause excessive knee extension and is potentially dangerous. Keep the knees soft and do not emphasise placing the heel on the floor when stepping back in L.I.A. patterns.

Lower Leg/Ankle/Foot

Footstrike patterns (both models are doing correct exercises)

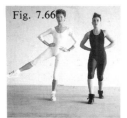

Pendulum/Stride

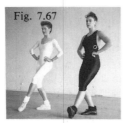

Toe point/Heel Jack

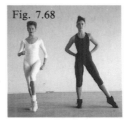

March/Step Touch

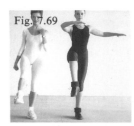

Flick Kick/Knee Lift

Repetitive stress

Lower leg pain and injuries to the ankle and foot are often the result of an excessive number of repetitions of the same foot strike pattern.

• Do no more than 32 consecutive footstrike patterns at one time.
• Do no more than 8 consecutive footstrike patterns on one leg (that is, no more than 4 hops or jumps on one leg) at a time.

• Do not do full tracks with one footstrike pattern (i.e. jogging on the spot) with only arm variations. Frequent foot pattern changes are most important to reduce impact stress.

Suggested footstrike patterns

Pendulum/stride (Figure 7.66), toe point/heel jack (Figure 7.67), march/step touch (Figure 7.68) and flick kick/knee lift (Figure 7.65).

The Sit-Up or the Crunch—Which is the Better?

There is an abundance of research that shows the strength gained from abdominal exercises can help prevent low back pain. However, recent evidence suggests that the type of abdominal exercise is also an important factor.

The straight leg sit-up's demise was instigated by research begun in the 1960s which showed that (a) when the legs are straight, the hip flexors and not the abdominals assume the major role in the exercise, and (b) anterior displacement of the fifth lumbar vertebra over the sacrum during the exercise could cause disc pressure problems.

The bent leg sit-up was proposed to get around this by putting the psoas and other hip flexors 'on the slack' thus reducing the adverse effects of their contraction. Still, electromyographical (EMG) studies have shown that the psoas is active in parts of the bent leg sit-up and this could even shorten and tighten the hip flexors because it involves them in a shorter range of motion (ROM).

The bigger potential problem is the intra-disc pressure found at the third lumbar disc by some Swedish researchers during a full bent leg sit-up. This was found to be about equal to that in forward flexion movements which are contra-indicated.

The Crunch

It has been shown that in either the bent leg or straight leg version of the sit-up, the abdominal muscles are essentially only used in the first third of the movement. So doing a full sit-up in either case is not warranted if abdominal strength is the objective.

A 'crunch', where the trunk is flexed no more than 30 degrees, is a better choice of exercise than a full sit-up (see the white model in Figures 7.28 to 7.32). These crunch exercises have been shown to recruit as many abdominal motor units as the full sit-up, but lack the potential disc pressure problems.

How Useful is the Inclined Sit-Up Board?

Little research has been done on the effectiveness of the sit-up board for working abdominal muscles. What has been done shows that these boards may be no more effective for the abdomen than working on a level surface. This is because trunk flexion with legs anchored primarily involves the hip flexor muscles, meaning that abdominals are probably used to no more than about 30% of their efficiency. Using a sit-up board with feet anchored is thought to have a similar effect.

Some manufacturers have attempted to overcome this by having boards where knees are bent over a knee rest. This causes other muscles (calves, hamstrings) to be involved in gripping the legs and, in effect, produces an effect similar to holding the feet down. An ordinary sit-up action from the floor with hips flexed and feet tucked under the buttocks still seems to offer the best of all worlds.

Back Extension Exercises

There are some 48 muscles in the region of the lower back alone, many of which are used infrequently. Sudden stress on these muscles can lead to problems, hence all exercises should be carried out correctly. Hyperextension of the lower back while lying prone with both arms and legs raised simultaneously, should be avoided.

A progression of safe exercises for strengthening the lower back while minimising strain is outlined below. While lying on the floor in the prone position (face down):

1. Lock the heels and buttocks together and hold 5–10 seconds, then relax. This tones some of the lower back muscles without placing any strain on the vertebral joints.

2. Progress to alternate leg lifts which strengthen the hamstrings and lower back.

3. To strengthen the muscles of the cervical and thoracic spine, place the hands behind the head and lift the head and shoulders. Cross the legs to prevent lifting them.

4. A progression of the above is to lift the shoulders and place the hands behind the back.

5. Progress to modified push-ups by raising only the head and shoulders and keeping the hips on the floor. (*Caution:* this should not be carried out by anyone with an excessive lordosis or 'sway back'.)

6. As an advanced exercise, place the hips over a pillow or bench and lift the legs alternately to a horizontal position.

Deep Knee Bends or Squats

When the knee is flexed beyond 90 degrees, the force on the joint can increase by up to 7 times body weight. This compression on the knee joint is exaggerated further if a weight is being lifted while in such a position. Pressure is put on part of the kneecap (patella) which is not well nourished. The result can be excessive wearing, and a 'click' as the joint surfaces slide past each other. Ultimately, there'll be knee pain.

On the other hand, the squat is one of the few exercises which incorporates the large muscles of the thighs in both heavy eccentric and concentric contractions. For this reason it resembles real-life sports actions more, probably, than any other quadriceps exercise. Changing one's stance from narrow to wide, toes in to toes out, and shifting weight from high on the shoulders to low on the shoulders or in front of the body, can vary the effort on the legs and back.

Taking everything into consideration, the conclusions of a National Strength and Conditioning Association forum on squatting are:

• If carried out correctly, the squat is one of the best compound exercises there is.

• The dangers of the full squat are in the execution of the exercise. Dangerous techniques include:
—Bouncing out of the bottom fully flexed position.
—Moving too quickly in the descent phase.
—Not keeping the centre of gravity over the middle of the feet.
—Carrying too much weight.
—Bending too far foward during the movement.
—Relaxing at the bottom of the squat before starting to stand up again.

• Although the full squat is probably not dangerous for the experienced when carried out correctly, there is little benefit in the beginner venturing anything deeper than the position of legs-parallel-to-the-floor.

• The depth of the squat should be determined by the purpose of the exercise. Quarter squats, for example, recruit muscles as in jogging. The parallel squat recruits muscles similar to sprinting and cycling.

• There may be some danger in adolescents squatting during a growth spurt (most likely 14–16 years) because of ligament 'looseness' which occurs at this age.

• While squatting to a bench may help define a safe range for the action, it could cause problems because of:
—Jarring of the spine and coccyx.
—The tendency to relax, then bounce out of the bottom position.
—A shift in body weight from bench to the beginning of the upward movement, causing strain.

The NSCA group also agreed on a number of points of technique in squatting with weights:

1. Face the squat rack when using weights rather than back in, so that the rack can be seen more safely after squatting.

2. Place feet apart shoulder-width or more.

3. Avoid excessive upper torso lean. Keep hips directly under the bar, head up.

4. Control the rate of descent to approximately 30 degrees per second.

5. Use 3 'spotters' if squatting with a heavy weight (one each side and one behind).

6. Keep feet flat on the floor (don't use a board under the feet). If flexibility isn't up to the job, develop it by gradually extending the depth of the squat.

7. Don't 'bounce' out of the bottom position: instead, accelerate out of it in order to use the quadriceps as much as possible.

8. Prevent the knees moving forward excessively during the action (they should be above the centre of the feet).

9. Individuals with weak backs, potential or confirmed, should use belts and ensure good form.

10. Avoid exhausting the abdominals and lower back before squatting as this can weaken the movement and lead to possible injury.

Back Pain

Statistics show that 8 out of 10 people will suffer some form of back pain at some stage of their lives, the most common area being the lower back, or lumbosacral spine.

This is hardly surprising as the back is used in almost all forms of activity—sitting, standing, bending, twisting, etc. As a result, many strains on the back are inevitable. Others can be avoided or lessened if the correct precautions are taken.

Anatomy of the Back

The spinal column consists of 24 movable bones and 7 less flexible ones (Figure 7.70). These are categorised into five areas as follows:

1. *Cervical* or neck vertebrae consisting of 7 bones.
2. *Thoracic* vertebrae, the 12 to the ribs.
3. *Lumbar* vertebrae are the largest and consist of 5 bones.
4. *The Sacrum* joins the spine to the pelvis. The sacrum is a wedge-shaped bone consisting of 5–7 fused vertebrae.
5. *Coccyx* or tail bone consisting of 2–4 fused vertebrae.

The vertebral column is like a string of beads which are separated by a thick fibrous structure called the intervertebral discs. These discs act as shock absorbers while also allowing for flexibility and movement of the spine in different directions.

The vertebral column is held together by strong ligaments and supported by muscles. With inactivity and age, the discs and ligaments may harden, leading to poor flexibility and eventually back pain.

Other reasons for back pain include:

1. Weak abdominal muscles due to a sedentary lifestyle and subsequent poor posture.
2. Weak back extensors, which again are due to lack of exercise and poor posture.
3. Tightening of the hamstring muscles from excessive running training in the absence of specific flexibility work.
4. Biomechanical factors such as leg length differences.

Exercises for the Back

The following exercises are designed to help you manage back trouble. It should be recognised, however, that these are only part of a wider approach to the problem. Learning how to lift correctly, stand, sit, and carry out other functional activities is vital if back pain is to be prevented or corrected. The ideal approach to back-care is a flexibility and strengthening program carried out in conjunction with yoga, tai-chai or other relaxation techniques.

Those already suffering back problems are advised to consult their doctor or physiotherapist, as exercise can aggravate certain types of back pain.

Cervical Spine or Neck Exercises

There are six basic movements of the neck:

• Flexion, or bending of the neck forward
• Extension or bending backwards
• Side flexion to the left and right
• Rotation of the head to the right and left.

All these can be combined in a single stretch movement by bending the head forward, rotating to

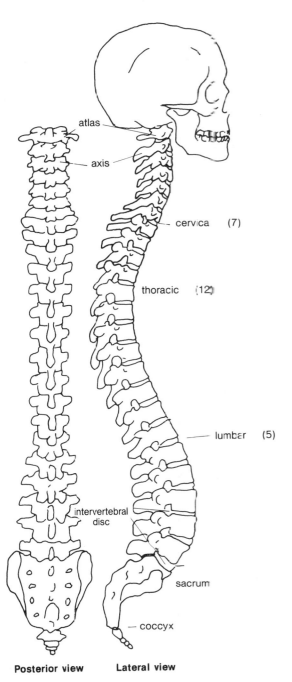

Fig. 7.70: Vertebrae and vertebral column

the side, then dropping the head back into extension, returning to the other side and finishing with the head on the chest. Direction can then be reversed.

Other neck stretches include tucking the chin and rotating the head (double chin exercise) and thrusting the neck forward and rotating the head (ostrich exercise). Isometric neck work can be done by resisting the movement of the neck with the palm of one or both hands.

Thoracic and Lumbar Spine

The following exercises aim to strengthen, mobilise and maintain maximum flexibility of the entire spine. Many are also excellent for improving posture in general. When doing these stretches go to the point of mild discomfort, hold for 15–30 seconds (longer if possible), then move into the stretch a little further.

1. *Spine Stretch (1):* Stretch hands above the head, 'think tall'.

2. *Spine Stretch (2):* Cross the arms and place the hands on the outside of the knees, pull the hands together and stretch up between the shoulder blades.

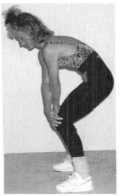
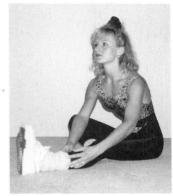

Fig. 7.71: Spine stretch (2)   Fig. 7.72: Spine stretch (3)

3. *Spine Stretch (3):* Move into a sitting position, reach forward, and clasp the hands behind the ankle.

4. *Spine Stretch (4):* Now sit with legs crossed. Place the hands on opposite knees and pull. This will stretch the upper spine.

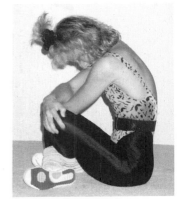

Figure 7.73: Spine Stretch (4)

5. *Shoulder Stretch:* Put right hand over right shoulder and left hand behind the back. Clasp fingers tightly and stretch, relax then repeat. Reverse arms and repeat the procedure.

6. *Head and Shoulder Raise:* Lie prone (face down) on the floor with hands behind the neck, raise head, hold, then relax.

7. *Opposite Arm/Leg Raise:* Lie prone on the floor and raise the opposite arm and leg slowly. Then repeat on the other side.

8. *Back Arch:* As above, except hands should be placed beside the body. As the head is raised, arms and shoulders should be stretched back.

9. *Spinal Ligament Stretch:* Lying on the back with the hands behind the head, raise the head upwards and forwards.

10. *Abdominal and Back Extensor Stretch:* Lie supine (face up) on the floor with knees bent. Push the lower back into the floor while breathing out; then, while breathing in, arch the spine upwards.

11. *Spinal Rotation:* Lying on the back, bend the right knee across the body and stretch the knee downwards with the left hand. Turn the head in the opposite direction.

12. *Hip and Knee Flexion Stretch:* Bend one knee up towards the body while lying on the back. Hold and hug with the arms. Alternate legs.

13. *Hip Hitching:* While lying prone, shorten one leg with respect to the other, then alternate legs.

14. *Cat-Arch Back Stretch:* Crouching on all fours, raise the spine slowly upwards, then relax.

15. *Alternate Arm/Leg Stretch:* While crouching on all fours, stretch the left hand above the head and right leg out behind, then alternate arms and legs.

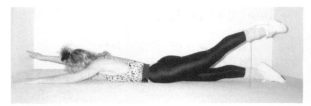
Fig. 7.74: Opposite arm/leg raise

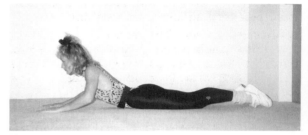
Fig. 7.75: Back arch

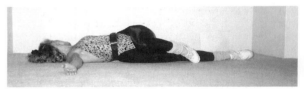
Fig. 7.76: Spinal rotation

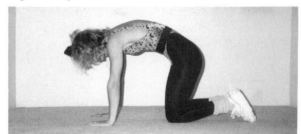
Fig. 7.77: Cat stretch

Exercise-Related Injuries

Injury due to physical activity can fall into three broad categories:

1. *Direct:* Includes sudden traumatic injuries such as 'cork thigh' which is caused by colliding with some object or person.

2. *Indirect:* Includes sprained ankles, pulled hamstrings etc., and is caused by excessive stress or strain on a muscle, ligament or joint.

3. *Overuse:* Includes many of the injuries suffered by instructors and participants. Examples of overuse injuries are shin splints, back pain and stress fractures.

Defining Injury Terms

Pain is nature's way of telling us that something is wrong. The location and severity of the pain can often indicate the type of injury that has been sustained.

1. *Muscle Strain* is a tear in the muscle-tendon complex. *Muscle spasms* are uncontrolled and painful muscle contractions which often occur as a protective mechanism after an injury has been sustained.

2. *Ligament Sprain:* The principal function of ligaments is to hold the bones together while the joint is moving. When ligaments are partially torn there is an inflammatory reaction causing swelling, pain and reduced movement.

3. *Tendinitis:* An inflammation of the tendon sheath as a result of over-use or biomechanical inefficiency. Tennis elbow is often a result of tendinitis.

4. *Haematoma:* A haematoma can occur as a result of damage to the blood vessels (bruising). If there is bleeding in interstitial tissue, and if it becomes clotted in the area of the injury, a haematoma may develop. If left untreated a calcium deposit could form.

5. *Stress Fractures:* Hairline breaks in a bone caused by overuse. If left unattended a shin splint can end up as a stress fracture to the tibia or fibula.

6. *Bursitis:* Bursae are closed sacs containing synovial fluid that are located in the body wherever there is a lot of friction and shock. Bursitis is an inflammation of the bursa.

Emergency First Aid for Injury

The immediate treatment for almost all exercise related injuries where the skin surface is not broken is the same, whether it is a pulled muscle, strained ligament, sore joint or a broken bone. This is a 5-part programme and is abbreviated as R.I.C.E.D.

R = Rest: Rest is necessary because continued activity could extend the injury.

I = Ice: Ice decreases the bleeding from the injured blood vessels through vaso-constriction. Ice may be applied every 2–3 hours for 15–20 minutes depending on the severity of the injury. Never use heat in the first 48 hours.

C = Compression: Compression limits the swelling which, if uncontrolled, could retard healing.

E = Elevation: Elevation of the injured part to above the level of the heart uses the force of gravity to help drain excess fluid.

D = Doctor: Consult a sports medicine specialist as soon as possible after the injury. Remember: early treatment speeds recovery and a quick return to activity.

8 Components of an Exercise Class

Aerobics to music was virtually unknown in the early 1970s. However, recently it has become one of the most popular forms of exercise, rivalling the more traditional programs such as jogging and swimming.

The word 'aerobic' has been used for years in the scientific world to describe the form of metabolism involving energy liberated in the muscle in the presence of oxygen. However, the term 'aerobics' has become synonymous in the public mind with exercise to music.

A good 'aerobics class' is in fact more than an aerobic program as it will include isolation strength work (anaerobic metabolism), flexibility, agility, co-ordination as well as providing a safe and social form of exercise.

The Structure of an Exercise Class To Music

The structure of an exercise class to music should be similar to that of other aerobic fitness programs, i.e. there should be a warm-up phase, a conditioning phase and a cool-down phase. The structure and dynamics of these phases is outlined below:

Sample Structure of an Exercise Class to Music

- Level of class: Intermediate
- Duration of class: 60 minutes
- Structure of Class: Single peak.

Phase 1 Warm-up

Purpose:
  i) Increase body temperature
  ii) Increase range of motion about the joints
  iii) Psychological preparation for the class

Duration: 10–15% of total class time (5–10 mins)

Intensity: Low to medium

Emphasis: Major muscles to be used in the class
  - Calves
  - Hamstrings
  - Chest
  - Quadriceps
  - Lower Back
  - Shoulders

Flexibility:
  Range of movement of major muscles
  Some static stretching of calves (optional)

Music:
  i) Style: Motivating and recognisable music
  ii) Speed: 128–138 bpm (intermediate class)

Exercises: Step touches, touch-backs with arm movements, side-steps, small lunges with arm movements and other LIA combinations.

Phase 2 Conditioning

Purpose:
  i) Aerobic conditioning
  ii) Muscular endurance

Duration: 75–80% of total class time (45 mins)
  i) Aerobic conditioning—30 mins
  ii) Muscular endurance—15 mins

Intensity: Medium to high

Emphasis:

i) Aerobic conditioning—keeping heart rate in training range i.e. between 65% and 80%

ii) Muscular endurance—isolate and overload the major muscle/muscle groups

Flexibility: Range of movement exercises are used at the end of the aerobic conditioning component prior to the commencement of the muscular endurance floor work

Music:

i) Style: Up tempo

ii) Speed:

Jumping tracks	—143 to 156 bpm
Run	—160 to 170 bpm
LIA	—133 to 144 bpm
Hi/low	—144 to 148 bpm
Muscular endurance	—100 to 126 bpm

Exercises:

i) Aerobic conditioning—Travelling combinations, step-touches, touch backs, heel touches, side leg kicks, lunges, knee lifts with hops and runs

ii) Muscular endurance—Abdominal curls, push ups, tricep dips, side leg lifts, back leg lifts, exercises for the upper and lower back.

Phase 3 Cool-Down

Purpose:

i) To prevent blood pooling

ii) To return the body to a steady state

iii) To stretch the muscles

Duration: 10% of total class time (6–10 mins)

Intensity: Low and decreasing to complete recovery

Emphasis:

i) Lower heart rate to resting level

ii) Stretch the major muscles

iii) Relaxation

Flexibility: Statically stretch the major muscles that have been used in the class with special emphasis on:

- Calves
- Quadriceps
- Shoulders
- Neck
- Shins
- Hamstrings
- Lower and Upper back

Music:

i) Style: Relaxing

ii) Speed: 110 bpm and below

Exercises: Static and PNF stretches.

The Warm-up

The purpose of the warm-up is to prepare the body for the conditioning phase of the class. There are three aspects to the warm-up:

i) Warming the body The prime function of this phase is to actually warm the body up. A general warming up can be achieved by using the major muscle groups in controlled, brisk, rhythmical activity. As the body heats up, the elasticity of the muscle is increased. Blood flow to the muscle is also increased enabling more oxygen to be carried to the muscles and facilitating the removal of waste products.

ii) Mobility Many class participants arrive with limited mobility due to sitting behind desks or driving for most of the day. Mobility can be achieved in conjunction with warming up movements by ensuring all joints are taken through a wide range of movement (ROM).

iii) Specific stretching This is a very contentious issue as some exercise scientists believe that static stretching should be a part of all warm-ups while others believe that ROM stretching is sufficient. A general consensus would suggest that static stretching be recommended for beginners or in a class where there is to be a high impact component (calves should be statically stretched) but it should only be done after a thorough warm-up.

The Conditioning Phase

This is the component that participants have come for so it must be dynamic. Instructors should structure the conditioning phase so that the desired target heart rate is achieved and there is sufficient overload on the major muscles while doing the floor work.

The *aerobic component* is aimed at improving the capacity of the body to delivery and use oxygen in the working muscles. To do this, the class should be sufficiently intense for the participants to reach a working heart rate of between 60% and 80% of maximum, for at least 20 minutes and preferably 30 minutes. The types of exercises selected should be those that incorporate large muscle groups: jumping, running, skipping, race walking, travelling moves and LIA steps are ideal. In all these movements the arms should be used to increase the intensity.

The Cool-Down Phase

This phase represents the tapering-off period after the completion of the conditioning phase. The aim is to return the body to a steady state. There are two aspects of this phase.

i) Recovery after the conditioning phase. This is best accomplished by a continuation of the conditioning phase at a decreasing intensity. This can be carried out by performing rhythmical movements similar to the warm-up or by the continuation of the isolation floor exercises. The intensity should decrease to a point

where the participants are only working on flexibility and relaxation exercises.

ii) Flexibility development This is essential at the conclusion of a class. Stretches should be static and held for at least 10 seconds. In addition PNF, partner and individual stretches can be incorporated into the cool-down.

Developing a Bank of Exercises

One of the greatest fears an instructor has when conducting a class is running out of exercises. Developing a large bank of effective exercises is therefore an important task for anyone wishing to become an exercise to music instructor.

There are four ways in which an instructor can vary an exercise:

1. Change the Lever

By changing the length of the lever (the arm or the leg) the instructor can generate numerous different exercises from one basic movement. When using *long levers* the intensity increases as the movement comes from the hip or shoulder joint. For example a flick kick, where the arms are moving from the shoulder in the full range of motion (see Figure 8.1(b)).

Short levers usually require flexion at the elbows and knees. This type of movement generally lowers the intensity level because of the more restricted range of motion (see Figure 8.1(a)).

2. Change the Plane

This is probably the most versatile way of developing new exercises. From one basic move the arm or legs can be changed to a horizontal, vertical or diagonal plane (see Figure 8.2), thereby giving the instructor a large array of exercises from one foot pattern. In addition, the instructor can vary the intensity depending on the plane chosen. For example, moving the arms from chest level to overhead can dramatically increase the intensity of the exercise.

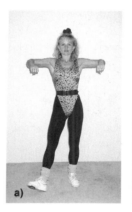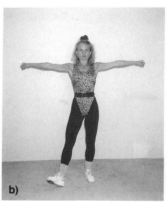

Fig. 8.1: Change the lever. Exercise (a) Short lever low intensity (b) Long lever high intensity

3. Change the Direction

By changing the direction the instructor can add variation to even the simplest moves. Travelling patterns such as moving forwards and backwards, from one side to the other, or diagonally across the floor vary the movement and also reduce impact stress. Direction can also be varied by changing the direction in which the body is facing.

Instructors should keep in mind that certain exercises travel in one direction better than others. For example, jumping jacks and other double foot jumping movements (which should be used in moderation) travel well backwards but not forwards.

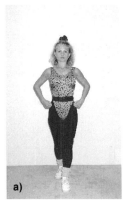
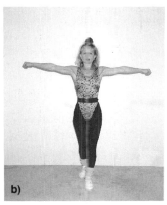
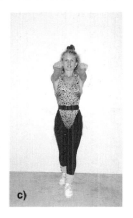
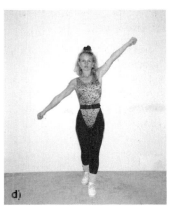

Fig. 8.2: Change the plane. (a) Start position—step back (b) Arms in horizontal plane (along the horizon) (c) Arms in vertical plane (up and down) d) Arms in diagonal plane (combination of both)

4. Change the Rhythm

Instructors can vary how much or how little movement occurs within a music phrase. There are three basic ways to vary the rhythm:

i) By the sound: get the participants to clap hands, click their fingers or stomp their feet
ii) By changing the repetitions: change the repetitions to either slow the exercise down or speed it up
iii) By the feel: encourage participants to feel 'crisp and staccato' or 'smooth and legato'. For example jumping jacks are crisp whereas letting the arms swing from one side to the other is smooth.

In addition to the above four ways of varying an exercise remember two golden rules:

1. For every foot pattern there are many arm variations
2. For every arm movement there are many foot variations.

Other ways of developing a bank of exercises are by:

• Attending other classes and naming any new exercises so that they can be remembered after the class
• Attending as many update and instructor training workshops as possible
• Reading fitness books and magazines
• Watching the latest exercise videos.

The above ideas are useless unless the instructor immediately rehearses any new exercises after seeing them, otherwise they will be forgotten very quickly.

Exercise Fluency and Transitions

Exercises that flow smoothly into one another make the class much easier to follow and more enjoyable for the participants. Furthermore, it assists the instructor in maintaining the intensity of the class thereby giving participants a more even workout.

When changing the plane of an exercise, the direction of an exercise or the lever used in an exercise always use *holding patterns* to ensure the transition is smooth.

Instructors should develop a series of holding patterns that they can always revert to when changing an exercise or, as can often happen, when the instructor

Aerobic track
↓
Low intensity LIA
↓
Range of movement for arms and legs
↓
Maintain arms while moving to the floor
↓
Commence floor work

Fig. 8.3: Fluency from an aerobic track to a floor track

has a mental block. Examples of simple holding patterns are:

• Jogging on the spot
• Step touch
• Standing leg raises
• Marching.

Another important time for fluency is moving down onto the floor after the aerobic component of the class (Figure 8.3). When moving from the floor to an aerobic track the same procedure should be used but in reverse.

Low Impact Aerobics

Injury prevention should be a primary consideration of all exercise to music instructors. The high incidence of anterior lower leg pain (often referred to as 'shin splints') can, in many instances, be attributed to high impact, repetitive foot strike movements. It is, therefore, important that instructors incorporate low impact moves into their aerobic tracks. This will reduce the stress caused by the high impact moves on the body's musculo-skeletal structure while still maintaining an aerobic training effect.

In addition to injury prevention LIA can be used:

i) to reduce the intensity of the track thereby making it ideal for beginners, older participants, the unfit and over weight.

ii) to add variety to the aerobic tracks

iii) to introduce participants to more complex dance moves

iv) to make transitions and to link different movement sequences.

LIA can be defined as a movement where one foot stays in contact with the ground most of the time. However, non-impact moves such as lunges, squats, plies also fall under the umbrella of LIA. LIA movements must have the potential to create a training effect. To accomplish this the large muscle groups of the thigh must be used. When lower body moves are combined with upper body movements, a training effect can be reached for exercisers of all fitness levels.

Low impact moves can be structured for the complete aerobic segment of the class, or alternating a low impact track with a high impact track. More commonly low impact moves are combined with high impact moves within the same track. Remember that for every high impact aerobic move there is a low impact version, and in many instances the exercise intensity will be much the same.

By performing an impact move, then following it with its low impact version, lower leg injuries can be reduced without reducing the overall training effect. For example, the high knee lift with the normal arm action. Repeat this eight times, then perform its low impact counterpart on the right leg four times. Repeat the standard high knee lift eight times then the low impact counterpart on the left leg 4 times (see Figure 8.4). This helps to make an interesting series of high/low moves out of one high impact move. Apply this technique to other moves and you are instantly choreographing simple routines.

Varying high impact with low impact moves is a hallmark of a well structured class. But instructors should be aware that there is a tendency for participants to excessively bend the knee of the supporting leg and place the trunk in a forward flexed position when doing LIA. This may lead to a different range of injuries than is caused by high impact exercises. Instructors should encourage participants to keep the back straight and not hyper-flex the knee.

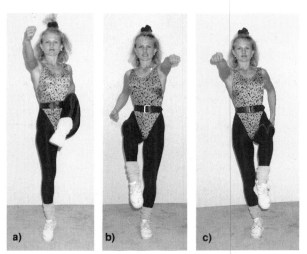

Fig. 8.4: (a) High impact knee lift (b) Low impact version on the right leg (c) Low impact version on the left leg

LIA Choreography

LIA basic moves consist of: step touch, push touch, low kick, knee lift, walking and twisting. To develop variations and create transitions from these basic LIA moves use the technique of: change the lever, change the plane, change the direction, change the rhythm and vary the intensity.

Table 8.1: Types of LIA tracks and ideal music speed

Type of LIA	Example	Speed of music
Stationary	• Non impact	138–152 bpm
	• Stationary steps	138–152 bpm
Travelling LIA	• Travelling sequences	138–144 bpm
	• Race walking	150–170 bpm
Combination	• High/low impact	144–148 bpm

Combinations

Developing combinations is a way an instructor can get the most out of different exercises. Any two similar movements can be added to form a combination of movements. Take for example the squat and the lunge.

Start the combination with the squat movement, using alternate bicep curls as the arm movement, for 16 counts followed by the lunge using the same arm movement. Once the participants know the 2 variations, repeat the moves for 8 counts then for 4 counts. This means the same movement can be repeated many times while still challenging the participants.

The same principle can also be applied to combinations using the same basic exercises (the squat and the lunge), e.g. repeat two different arm movements with the same squat or lunge movements, or use the same arm movement with a combination of dynamic squat or lunge exercise.

Simply stated then, building combinations involves putting patterns together. The combination can be as uncomplicated as using one base movement with two elements of variation or it can be more challenging using two different base steps such as a jumping jack and skip.

Organised Action

The traditional aerobic class format consisted of an individual staying in one spot and working out in isolation from the other participants. Fortunately, there is an abandonment of this 'no contact', 'don't leave your spot' philosophy, as more and more instructors have begun to promote a variety of group activities among class participants. Included in this category of 'organised action' are circuits, formations, partner work, relays and other types of group activities.

In all forms of 'organised action' there are a series of common organisation principles. One essential factor is adequate instructor preparation and rehearsal so the complex routine involving numbers of people does not break down into a disorganised mess. Besides taking into account such factors as adequate spacing,

appropriate music, etc, the instructor should also ensure that the class participants are aware of what they will be doing. For example, pre-class instruction might include partners pairing off at that time, circuit teams being organised or class participants being numbered in a team system that will be employed later in the class.

Line Work Formations

Line work formations are basically self explanatory (see Figure 8.5). One consideration is to be certain to divide the class up evenly, perhaps even employing a numbering system developed during the pre-class instruction.

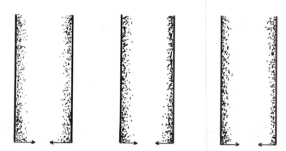

1. With 6 lines: Each pair of lines faces each other and does a set movement

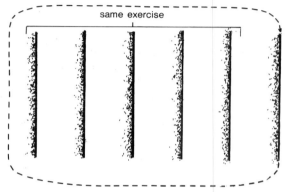

2. With 6 lines: All lines do the same exercise and one line runs around the rest

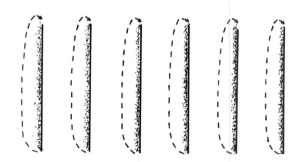

3. With 6 lines: Each individual line runs around its own line

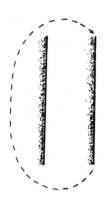

4. With 2 lines: Both lines face each other and mirror each other's movements. Or, one line runs around the other.

Fig. 8.5: Organised Action lines

Circle Activities

When doing circle work it is advisable that the instructor moves in the opposite direction to the group as this promotes a more effective teaching position (see Figure 8.6).

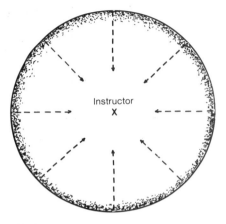

Fig. 8.6: Circles. One large circle around the instructor. Circle moves towards the instructor and then moves back. Or participants race walk around the room doing different arm exercises. The instructor should always move in the opposite direction.

Circuits

A variety of circuits can quite easily be devised for inclusion in the class. The most easily implemented circuit is the free style circuit in which no equipment is necessary (see Figure 8.7).

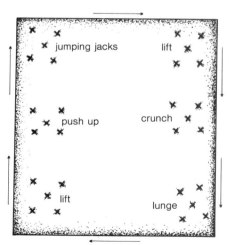

Fig. 8.7: Circuits. The instructor is usually only limited by his/her imagination

Exercise Cueing

Effective exercise cueing can be what distinguishes the good from the average instructor. The reason being that class participants always follow the instructor's first movement, and if it is wrong, the fluency of the class is lost and the instructor loses credibility. It is important, then, that the instructor always uses good cueing techniques when changing from one exercise to another.

Cues may be defined as verbal or non verbal:

Verbal

• Direction or placement—tells where to go
• Countdown/timing—how many to go and when to change
• Technique/quality—signal change in intensity, pace and rhythm

• Intonation—helps reinforce, particularly quality cues and power words
• Praise or progress—lets participants know how they are doing
• Exercise vocabulary—words, phrases and imagery can tell what, how much and when.

Non verbal

• Signs or symbols—hand signals or cards etc.
• Facial expressions—eye contact etc.
• Music—contains built in cues that are in rhythm, phrasing and lyric composition
• Exercise selection and progression—logical and simple steps make cueing easier
• Props—whistles, tambourines, cue cards, circuit cards.

Class Structures and Strategies

Over the past 10 years exercise to music classes have developed so rapidly that scientific investigation of physiological effects and methods of organisation has lagged behind development. While it is generally agreed that exercises to music can change aerobic capacity, there has been very little investigation into the consequences of sequencing or formatting of exercises within an exercise class.

In 1988, Paul Batman from the Sydney Institute of Education examined in detail the physiological responses to different class formats. The specific class formats studied were as follows:

1. Single peak format consisting of warm-up, LIA (travelling) jump, run, LIA (stationary), floor work followed by a cool-down

2. Reverse peak format consisting of warm-up, floor work, LIA (stationary), run, LIA (travelling) followed by a cool-down

3. Multi-peak format consisting of warm-up, LIA (travelling), LIA (stationary), jump, floor work, run, floorwork followed by cool-down

4. Continuous multi-peak format consisting of the multi-peak sequence repeated twice.

The results of the investigation revealed that exercises to music classes using any one of the four formats produced heart rates high enough to facilitate an aerobic training effect. An examination of the mean heart rates for all formats showed that all movement tracks produced heart rates in excess of 70% of maximum heart rates. This research would then indicate that the format of the class is not a limiting factor to aerobic metabolism. So what then is recommended format? The answer is simple: the format that the instructor feels the most comfortable with. Table 8.2 outlines the advantages and disadvantages of each format.

Table 8.2: The advantages and disadvantages of different class structures

Advantages	Disadvantages
1. Multi-peak	
• Good variety	• Transitions down to the floor and up again are challenging
• Good for beginners	• Transitions are time consuming
• Less stress on the lower leg	• If not well thought out, class can have an irregular flow
• Stops burn-out at the end of the aerobic tracks	• Harder to isolate muscles in the floor tracks
• Good for men and athletes	• Requires an experienced teacher
• Instructors do not need as large a bank of exercises	

Advantages	Disadvantages	Advantages	Disadvantages

2. Single peak

- Easy to achieve target heart range in the aerobic segment
- Intensity is consistent
- High energy levels attained in the aerobic segment
- Less transitions so easier to organise
- Good for isolating muscle groups in the floor work
- The body is well warmed up for the floor work
- Good for overloading class participants

Disadvantages (col 2):
- Fatigue during the aerobic segment may result in poor form or technique in both aerobic segment and floor work
- Continuous high stress placed on the lower legs
- Very predictable—less variety
- Difficult for beginners to maintain the required intensity in the aerobic segment
- Can reinforce the myth of spot reduction

3. Reverse peak

- Many of the same advantages as the single peak
- Adds variety
- With the floor work finished participants may put more energy into the aerobic segment
- Body well warmed up for the static stretching in the cool-down.

Disadvantages (col 4):
- The body may not be warmed up for the floor work
- The time required for the cool-down needs to be extended
- The time for the aerobic segment may need to be reduced.

4. Dual or continuous multi-peak

- Good for beginners
- Reduces impact stress
- Allows for a good break up of the aerobic segment

Disadvantages:
- Insufficient overload for advanced participants
- The many transitions required are time consuming and reduce intensity.

Music: The Key to Successful Exercise Classes

One of the most important elements of a successful class is the music. However, prior to selecting the music for the class the following decisions must be made:

- What type of class is going to be taught? Will it be a single peak, multi-peak or reverse peak class?
- What level of tempo should be selected? Will the tempo correspond with the class type and participant needs?
- Who will the participants be? Will they be housewives, teenagers, sports people, business types, school children?
- What mood or style is to be used? Will the participants prefer radio hits, classic tracks, rock or disco?

Once the above decisions have been made then each track can be planned and the speed and type of music selected. The speed of music refers to the beats per minute (bpm). To determine the bpm first establish the base beat. Then count the number of beats in 15 seconds, multiply this by 4 and you have the bpm (see Table 8.3).

The warm-up is the opening track and therefore must be inspiring and energising. A bad choice here can put a damper on the class.

The music selection and tempo for the aerobic segment must vary depending on whether the track is to be a run, a jump or LIA. Running at speeds that

Table 8.3 Suggested BPM Chart

Component of class	Music beats per minute (BPM)
• Warm-up	128–135
• Jump	148–156
• Run	160–174
• LIA	134–144
• High/Low	144–148
• Floor	100–126
• Isolation Weights	100–116
• Travelling Weights	120–130
• Cool-down	110–and below

are too slow, say 150 bpm, feels awkward and detracts from the effectiveness of the track. On the other hand a tempo of 160 beats for LIA is far too fast as it will affect range of motion and hence the form of the participants.

Music selection for the cool-down should be of a slow tempo and relaxing. It is one of the easiest tracks to plan as there is plenty of suitable music around.

Recording Tips

- Access to a variable speed turntable will enable you to vary the speed of the record to suit the planned track.

- Ensure that the heads on the tape deck are clean otherwise the clarity of the recording will be affected.
- Check the recording level of each song otherwise your tape will play back at different volumes.
- Record the floorwork and cool-down at a lower level so that you do not have to adjust the volume in the class.
- Always use good quality tapes. It is obvious to the participants when the instructor uses a cheap tape.

Additional Points for the Instructor

Lower Back Problems

Most people at some stage suffer from lower back problems as a result of either poor posture, weak back extensors, tight hamstrings or weak abdominal muscles.

Back injuries tend to recur and can often be aggravated by exercise. This is especially so with exercises that use the lumbar/sacrum as a fulcrum with no support, and those using hyper-extension of the lower back. Instructors should be aware of the dangers when the lower back is placed in a *forward flexed* and unsupported position.

The guidelines for forward flexion in an exercise to music class are as follows:

i) Never be in a forward flexed position with locked knees
ii) Never do forward flexion with spinal rotation
iii) Never do forward flexion with speed
iv) Never go beyond 30 degrees in a forward flexed position when unsupported
v) Never hang in a forward flexed position whether supported or unsupported for more than 15 seconds
vi) Forward flexion when kneeling is also contra-indicated.

The above guidelines may seem restrictive but there are many safe back exercises that can be substituted for those that incorporate forward flexion. Instructors who are unsure about the safety of an exercise, especially if it incorporates forward flexion, are advised to remove it from their routine and replace it with a recognised safe exercise.

Legal Liability

It is imperative that instructors take adequate care to prevent injury to their class participants. However, all the care in the world does not prevent accidents from happening. Avoiding liability is impossible. For example, in the middle of a running track someone is accidentally 'tripped up' and falls and breaks an arm. It is the instructor who is responsible, not the person who did the tripping. Put simply, an instructor cannot avoid being liable no matter how careful she or he is.

Instructors who work for a large fitness centre cannot afford to trust the 'deep pocket theory'. This refers to the theory that lawsuits are only filed against the party with the most money. Be warned that all parties named in a lawsuit are united under a legal term known as 'joint and several' liability. This means that all defendants named in a lawsuit are collectively responsible for the damages.

Professional Indemnity

Professional indemnity means that the instructor is protected if a participant is injured or dissatisfied and he/she claims the instructor was responsible. In some cases the claim may be that the instructor was being unprofessional by exposing them to potentially harmful exercises. In other cases it may simply be based on an accident or mishap which occurred during the class or at the venue.

Professional indemnity insurance is different to public liability. Public liability covers the fitness centre in the event that an accident occurs in the facility. For example, a club member may slip in the wet area of the centre and break a leg. Public liability will cover this mishap, not professional indemnity.

In Australia professional indemnity is available to professional fitness instructors and those instructors who are registered by a recognised certifying authority. Professional associations can provide professional indemnity insurance cover for fitness instructors and centre operators

Lactic Acid and the Exercise Class to Music

The term 'anaerobic' refers to the production of energy in the absence of oxygen. The major drawback of anaerobic glycolysis (glycolysis refers to the breakdown of sugar) is that the sugar is only partly broken down. This results in the accumulation of lactic acid.

The primary objective of the floorwork component of an exercise class is to improve muscular endurance. Muscular endurance is the ability of a muscle to exert force against a given resistance without total fatigue. To achieve this improvement the muscles must be overloaded beyond their normal capacity with a slight accumulation of lactic acid. As muscles become conditioned through anaerobic work they develop a greater tolerance to lactic acid and can function longer. This in turn can improve aerobic fitness by allowing you to train harder and longer.

Although a slight accumulation is favourable, in excess it can have a number of negative consequences. It can cause discomfort, temporary fatigue, feelings of nausea, poor form and feelings of inadequacy. As such it is important that aerobic instructors have an understanding of the positive and negative effects of the accumulation of lactic acid.

Exercise nausea

Excessive accumulation of lactic acid can cause feelings of nausea. Beginners or deconditioned people are particularly prone to producing high blood lactate levels quickly, more so if doing an intermediate or advanced class. Instructors should demonstrate modified exercises and encourage new exercisers to work at their own pace and not compete with other participants or try to keep up with the instructor.

Accumulation in supporting muscles

During floorwork, instructors should include transition exercises to help reduce fatigue. Take for example a lateral leg lift where one leg is supporting the body and the other is being exercised. If the instructor immediately changes legs and begins working the support leg, it will fatigue very quickly. Participants compensate for this by changing their body alignment which can compromise the safety of the back.

To prevent the support leg being over-fatigued the instructor should include a transition exercise that works an unrelated muscle or muscle group.

Avoid excessive repetitions

Instructors should not use their own feelings of fatigue as a yardstick as to how the class participants are feeling. The instructor should always be 'fitter' than most of the participants and what may be easy for the instructor could be 'total burnout' for the participants. In order to prevent this the instructor should bear in mind two things. The first is to avoid excessive repetitions as this unnecessarily fatigues the muscle or muscle group. The second is to have a large bank of exercises for each muscle or muscle group to ensure variation.

Accumulation during abdominal exercises

Often in an 'abdominal' track, an excessive number of crunches and crunch variations are performed. Individuals may experience excessive overload in their abdominal muscles. Instructors can compensate for this by encouraging those participants who are fatiguing to raise their buttocks off the ground every few crunches (Figure 8.8). This movement involves contraction of the erector spinae and gives the abdominals a chance to stretch and relax. The blood flow to the abdominal muscle increases and assists in the removal of lactic acid.

Relationship of lactic acid to travelling and jumping moves

Even though travelling and jumping tracks are structured to develop aerobic capacity they can sometimes be too intense and place the less fit participants in oxygen debt. To prevent this, instructors should intersperse low impact variations during high impact moves. In addition, beginners should be encouraged to use the low impact variation if they find the high impact move too fatiguing.

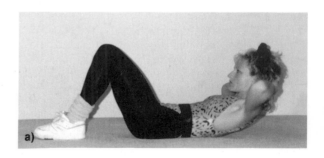

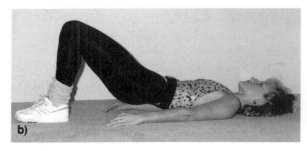

Fig. 8.8: a) Abdominal crunch
b) Relaxation of abdominals

Does lactic acid cause muscle soreness?

A common belief is that the accumulation of lactic acid is the primary cause of post exercise muscle soreness. This soreness is often felt 24–48 hours after unfamiliar or overly strenuous exercise. However, the removal of lactic acid from the blood and muscle is fairly rapid. After maximal exercise almost 95% is removed in about one hour. This recovery can be accelerated by doing light rhythmical exercise. Therefore, lactic acid is not considered to be the cause of post exercise soreness. The most commonly accepted theory is the minute muscle tears that result from the eccentric phase of muscle contraction.

Lactic acid needn't be viewed as the 'aerobic exerciser's enemy'. In fact it's a vital part of the conditioning process. However, its accumulation does need to be controlled and this is simply done with a bit of understanding and planning. Keep an eye on your participants. If they stop exercising or their form changes it's likely that they are truly suffering from fatigue. Move on to another muscle group and return if you wish. By then they'll be ready for another round.

Advice for Floor Class Instructors

To improve floor class programs the instructor can:

1. Talk to participants during the class, giving encouragement and singling out various points of an exercise being carried out.

2. Encourage members to work to their own ability and not to compete with others in the class or with the instructor.

3. Encourage beginners to do some of each exercise at a reduced rate rather than try to keep up until they can no longer continue.

4. Explain the reasons for doing an exercise in a particular way and particularly the need for warm-up and cool-down periods.

5. Take the trouble to find out a participant's sporting interests and emphasise any specific exercises in the class that could be of benefit for that sport.

6. Be aware of the muscles involved in each exercise and the major muscles and energy systems used in the class.

7. Encourage high quality work from everyone rather than the specific involvement of just a few. An instructor will earn no respect by competing with the fittest participant.

8. Show some vitality, understanding and humour. Exercise should be fun as well as satisfying an important function.

The Freelance Instructor

Freelance instructing has become a regular and exciting way of earning income for many fitness exponents. There are three main areas where a living can be earned:
- Health and fitness centres
- In-house programs in business and industry
- Community centres, halls and sporting clubs.

Each requires a different approach and a different attitude on the part of the instructor. For example:

Health and Fitness Centres

For many this is the start. The policies of an individual centre must be respected, but an aspiring teacher can become familiar with style, music, reaction of the clients and their expectations of the instructor by simply observing or participating in regular classes.

Discussions with management are necessary to determine the types of exercises; music (yours or theirs); music volume; dress regulations; client contact; fees and collection.

Centres provide the ideal situation for learning. But the following words of warning should be heeded:
- Don't expect to re-educate clients, and particularly management. Habits are hard to change.
- Be prepared for lack of acceptance from clients; they get attached to certain styles and instructors.
- Don't work at a centre where methods and policies are suspect.

In-house Programs in Business and Industry

This is becoming a growth area as more and more organisations realise the value of a fit workforce. Many organisations can provide a ready class of 15–50 people either before or after regular work hours or during the lunch break. Some organisations even provide time off work for staff exercise.

Often the main limitation to the class in the workplace is space. However, with access to showers, portable mats and a portable cassette deck, only a limited space is necessary.

In negotiating fees and time for in-house programs, management should be dealt with directly. Personal contacts are also best for establishing classes in various businesses. Fees can be charged on a per person basis or as a set fee per class and the organisation can either be invoiced or a members' committee appointed to collect fees.

All participants should be screened before commencing an in-house program and advice should be provided on monitoring individual improvement. As with set classes it is important to provide regular feedback to clients to ensure continued interest.

Community Centres, Halls and Sporting Clubs

This type of enterprise differs from the first two in that there are personal overheads, and the general public will be involved. More than likely it will be necessary to rent space, advertise and take out insurance for professional indemnity.

Before opening private classes, a thorough market search of the area should be carried out to determine what other classes exist, their times and cost. A target market should be selected (i.e. women, older people, housewives, etc.) and promotions aimed specifically at that group.

Locations that may be suitable include council rooms; church/masonic/school halls; police citizens' boys' clubs; RSL, Leagues clubs; golf, bowling clubs; squash centres.

In many instances it is possible to negotiate a rental fee based on percentage of earnings, at least in the early stages while clientele is building up. A review can be made after 6 months, when a flat fee may be more acceptable.

Point-of-sale advertising (posters, signs, etc.) are often the best form of advertising, but notices can also be placed in local libraries, baby health centres, dentists' and doctors' surgeries, laundromats, shops, banks, hairdressers etc. Leaflets can also be left or displayed in all of the above-mentioned locations. Because of the expense and the regularity required, newspaper advertising is probably not a good form of promotion for the freelance.

Records of all receipts and expenses should be kept diligently, and if possible an accountant or bookkeeper used to keep accounts. An insurance agent should also be consulted about personal accident and sickness insurance.

Finally, some pointers on setting up:

• Don't overcrowd your timetable. Administration and promotional aspects are also time-consuming.
• Don't spread yourself too thin—too many classes can cut down your productive life.
• Don't rely totally on a fitness income when starting. This should be aimed at as a longer term goal.

Exercises in Confined Spaces

For this section a 'confined space' is defined as a floor area that accommodates a minimum of 10 persons and a maximum of 30, that is, a floor area of approximately between 22.5 m² (220 sq. ft.) and 67.5 m² (620 sq. ft.). This is using a base of 2.25 m² (20 sq. ft.) per person and an extra equal space (2.25 m²) for the instructor.

Looking at exercises in confined spaces it is of course necessary to first determine what is to be accomplished. For the purposes of this discussion we'll address ourselves to aerobic exercises which look to increase flexibility, endurance and cardiovascular efficiency.

When first looking at a small room where exercises are to be performed it is easy to become discouraged. Don't be constricted when looking at any space, as this may close off certain possibilities. It is more difficult to work in a small space than a large one, especially with a particularly fit class, but it can be done and it can be rewarding.

Guidelines for Running Floor Classes

1. The class must include a warm-up phase (5–10 minutes); a conditioning phase (at least 15 minutes); a cool-down phase (5–10 minutes).

2. Music should be selected to allow for a good general warm-up at a gentle rate before more strenuous work is carried out.

3. No entry onto the floor should be allowed after the warm-up has started. A safe, professionally structured class cannot be run properly if members are allowed to begin in dribs and drabs.

4. Well-cushioned shoes should be compulsory. Running or jumping in bare feet, even on carpeted areas, can cause bruised heels, sore calf muscles and contribute to other injuries like shin splints.

5. Participants should be encouraged to attend floor classes or carry out some other form of aerobic exercise at least 3 days a week.

6. As far as possible classes should be structured to cater at least for beginning and advanced exercisers (preferably with an intermediate level), with separate classes conducted for each.

7. Stretching should be static or PNF and should include the major muscle groups to be used in the exercise to follow.

8. All new participants in a class should be questioned as to their previous exercise levels and advised as to the level recommended for their purpose.

9. Participants should be advised from the start of the program as to how long the class will be, and of any idiosyncracies of the class that may not be expected.

10. Participants must be asked if they are taking any form of medication, and if so what this is. Where no knowledge about a medication is immediately available, steps should be taken to ascertain contra-indications of exercise, if any.

11. Participants should be advised to exercise before rather than after eating, but that limited fluid intake (with the exception of alcohol) before (and even during) extended exercise is advisable.

12. Exercise involving deep knee bends, forward flexion or hyperextension of the lower back should be avoided.

13. Attention must be given to the correct procedures in carrying out exercises, e.g. sit-ups should be done with legs bent, leg raises with some back support, etc.

14. Advice should be given to certain participants about the level of difficulty of some exercises, e.g. many men may have difficulty with certain flexibility exercises more suited to women (adductor/abductor stretches, back flexes, etc.).

15. Precaution must be taken at all times to prevent both acute and chronic injury. This includes caution against the over-use of certain techniques such as bouncing on toes, or running with bare feet on hard surfaces.

16. Ideally, one other instructor should be on the floor assisting the instructor taking the class. His/her job is to correct exercises and give advice and encouragement, particularly for beginners.

17. Participants should be asked to remove watches, jewellery and other accessories that may interfere with the full range of movement of an exercise.

18. Clothing should be loose fitting to allow proper freedom of movement. Plastic suits, wraps, etc. should not be allowed on the floor. Heavy track suits and leg warmers may be worn for the warm-up, but should then be discarded to prevent over-heating.

19. Ballistic type stretching is not advisable.

20. Instructors should have a current first aid certificate including knowledge of cardiopulmonary resuscitation (CPR). A good first aid kit and instant ice packs should also be readily available in the unlikely event of an accident. An emergency phone number should also be close handy.

21. Floor areas should not be overcrowded. Crowding restricts the range of exercises that can be carried out and makes running difficult if not dangerous.

22. Ensure the exercise space is well ventilated and try to keep the temperature relatively cool, at between 15–20 degrees C. Cold air from an air conditioner or open window should be avoided.

9 Aquafitness

Aquafitness (sometimes called 'Waterobics', 'Aquarobics', 'Hydro-exercise' etc.) is the term used to describe a variety of exercises, circuits, games and dances performed in water. Aquafitness is based on two fundamental properties of water:

- That it is a buoyant medium
- That it exerts resistance to motion.

Neither of these forces apply on land.

Aquafitness is a viable alternative to land-based exercise and the home pool provides an ideal facility for an Aquafitness program. Water exercise has wide appeal and has proved popular with people who may not have otherwise been involved in exercise.

Benefits

The benefits of exercising in water have been well known since Greek and Roman times. Water exercise has a number of benefits over land based work, e.g.:

1. Exercising in water is easier: it supports body weight (up to 85% in water to up to chest level).

2. Water acts as a shock absorber, reducing the stress on joints.

3. Water exerts resistance to motion. The degree of resistance depends on the speed and manner in which the movement is performed.

4. Provided the temperature is appropriate for the type of class, the risk of over-heating is reduced as the water acts as a coolant.

5. Water allows a full range of movement without excessive strain. Yet less co-ordinated individuals can carry out movements in water without the embarrassment they may feel with ordinary exercises.

6. There is little post-exercise stiffness. This is due, possibly, to lack of eccentric muscular contractions combined with the decreased muscle tone experienced in water.

7. The massage effect of water increases circulation and promotes relaxation.

8. Aquafitness is a novel and enjoyable way to become and stay fit.

Safety Factors

Some important safety considerations are:

1. A momentary rise in blood pressure occurs when a person enters the water. Immersion should be gradual.

2. There is a risk of hypothermia if body heat is lost too quickly during or immediately following exercise in pools with a temperature below 25 degrees C, and

a risk of hyperthermia where the temperature is above 30 degrees C.

3. Pool chemicals should be maintained at strictly correct levels to prevent the risk of infection or skin irritation. Showering and using moisturiser after the class are recommended, as is the use of anti-fungal powder on the feet.

4. Teaching correct form is essential as close individual monitoring of an Aquafitness class is difficult, e.g.:

• Avoid the natural inclination to jog and jump on the toes whilst in the water. Use the whole foot in order to avoid cramp or leg injury.

• Whenever performing stomach strengthening exercises with the back against the pool wall, be sure the pelvis is tilted forward.

5. When demonstrating on the pool-side, wear adequate protective footwear or use a gym mat or mini-trampoline.

6. Where possible, use non-verbal communication to save vocal cords.

7. Knowledge of first aid, cardio-pulmonary resuscitation and water rescue techniques is essential.

Venue Requirements

The following should be available in a good venue:

• Correct depth of water, waist to chest deep
• Correct water temperature
    25°C Aquarobics
    28°C Pre- and post-Natal
    33°C Stretch & Movement
• Non-slip pool surrounds and floor
• Ramp or steps for entry and exit
• A rail, ledge or gutter at water level
• Sufficient areas around the pool for the instructor to demonstrate.

Programming for Aquafitness

Aquafitness classes should follow the same general guidelines as any other program. The class should include a warm-up, conditioning and cool-down phase, keeping in mind that within these parameters there are a number of variables which can be changed such as the depth of water, the speed of the exercises or the amount of turbulance created. The instructor can also use different kinds of music and equipment (balls, hoops, inner tubes, flippers etc.) to add variety.

Target Groups

One of the main benefits of an Aquafitness program is that all age-groups and fitness levels can participate. Some of the groups for whom the activity is suitable are:

    Athletes
    Injured athletes
    Children
    Pre- & post-natal mothers
    Overweight people
    Older adults
    Frail aged
    Disabled—physically and intellectually

Guidelines for some of these groups are considered below, individually. General guidelines for the running of Aquafitness classes are given at the end of the chapter.

Athletes

Programs for athletes are usually planned specifically to improve performance in a particular sport or activity. Some of their special needs are considered below.

Profile of the athlete:

• High aerobic fitness
• Good muscle tone/strength
• Motivated
• Often poor flexibility
• Co-ordination could be improved
• Often stressed.

Guidelines:

1. Capitalise on the resistance properties of water. Include handboards, weights and flotation devices.

2. Use deepwater techniques to increase difficulty and aerobic effect.

3. Include circuit training.

4. Work on flexibility and co-ordination.

5. Encourage relaxation.

Children

Programs for children are often run as part of the school curriculum these days. The objective may be to build water confidence as part of a learn-to-swim program or as an alternative to competitive sport, with the emphasis on social development and learning through play.

Under-12 years profile:
• High lean tissue/fat ratio causes children to lose body heat rapidly.
• Able to perform tasks suited to their stage of development.
• Can be at various levels of water confidence.

Guidelines:
1. Water should be heated (25 degrees C).
2. Water should be no deeper than chest height.
3. Exercises should be simple to understand, short in duration, and fun.
4. Add variety by including equipment in class (e.g. hoops, rings, balls, inner tubes etc.).
5. Exercises can include simple variations on themes of movement, including:

• Walking in circles	• Jumping-jacks
• Bunny hops	• Marching
• Jogging	• Dancing
• Hopping	• Games etc.

Pre- and Post-Natal Women

Aquafitness is recommended by many doctors for pregnant women because in water they are not disadvantaged by their condition or extra size. When prescribing such a program it is important to remember that pregnancy is a healthy state, not a 'medical condition'!

Profile of the pre- and post-natal woman:
• Increased heart rate and cardiac output
• Increased core temperature
• Increased breast size may lead to fibrous tissue breakdown which is irreversible
• A special hormone, 'relaxin', is released to loosen the joints in the pelvic area. This can have a weakening effect on joints
• Postural changes can lead to lower back pain if care is not taken
• In about 30% of women the linea alba between the rectus abdominus muscles may soften and weaken
• About 30% of women who have never had children and 80% of pregnant women experience a weakening of pelvic floor muscles which can cause incontinence.
• As pregnancy progresses, circulation in the lower limbs becomes impaired, often leading to severe cramping.

Guidelines:
1. Check on the participant's general amount of exercise undertaken during pregnancy.
2. Work at a maximum level of 70% MHR.
3. Avoid over-heated pools (over 30 degrees C) for pre-natal classes.
4. Adequate breast support is essential during exercise.
5. Key skeletal muscles should be strengthened to compensate for the change in centre of gravity. In particular these are:

> abdominals
> gluteals
> hip flexors
> extensors of the spine and neck.

6. Check for separation between the abdominal muscles by placing fingers between the bands of recti muscles when the woman is lying in the supine position with chin raised. Three or more fingers' width indicates a need for a gentle abdomen-strengthening program.

7. Include pelvic floor exercises.

8. Avoid exercises involving toe pointing as these can precipitate leg cramp. Add exercises to increase circulation in lower limbs, such as calf stretch, ankle circles etc.

9. Advise pregnant participants to eat complex carbohydrate 1 hour prior to a class in order to avoid fatigue and dizziness. Encourage a well-balanced diet.

Older Adults

Much of the growth in popularity of Aquafitness classes has been due to the interest of older adults who find such classes fun, easy to do, and not physically stressful on aged joints.

Profile of the older adult:
• Often have weak muscles
• A tightening of postural muscles and weakening of

phasic muscles with age can lead to increased lower back problems
• Freedom of movement can be restricted due to joint deterioration and swelling caused by arthritis
• Poor diet, malabsorption of nutrients and changes in hormone levels can lead to brittle bones
• Gradual loss of proprioceptive sensitivity in the feet affects sense of position, balance and body awareness
• Around 60% of older women may have weak pelvic floor muscles which can affect bladder control, causing incontinence
• Possible heart and circulatory disorders
• Often on medication.

Guidelines:
1. Focus on gentle exercise.
2. Ensure water temperature is between 28–33° C.
3. Focus on body awareness, balance, co-ordination, flexibility and strength.
4. Avoid grinding repetitive movements which can cause injury.
5. Include pelvic floor exercises.
6. Teach heart rate monitoring and its purpose (use radial not carotid pulse).
7. Discourage participants with heart conditions from exercising with their arms above their heads.
8. Check medication and its effect during exercise.

Aquafitness Exercises

The following is a sample of body positions, stretches and exercises which are used in the water. Others can be adapted from the ones used on land.

Body Positions

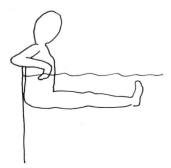

Fig. 9.1: Back braced

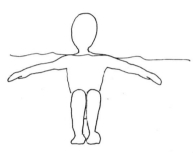

Fig. 9.2: Sit float

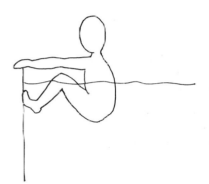

Fig. 9.3: Backstroke start

Stretches

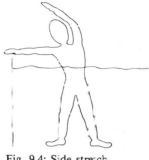

Fig. 9.4: Side stretch

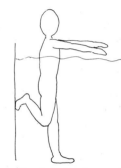

Fig. 9.5: Quad stretch

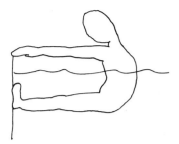

Fig. 9.6: Universal stretch
(hamstring, back, shoulders)

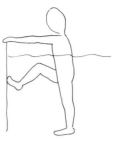

Fig. 9.10: Pool wall step-ups

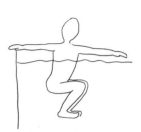

Fig. 9.11: Side tucks

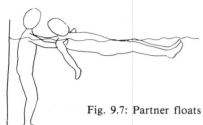

Fig. 9.7: Partner floats

Exercises

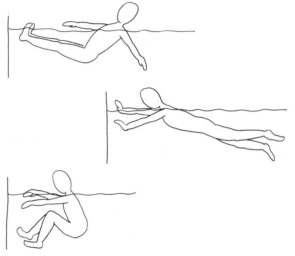

Fig. 9.12: Water burpies (leg extensions, knee tucks,
backwards kicks)

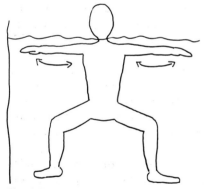

Fig. 9.8: Backward and forward flies

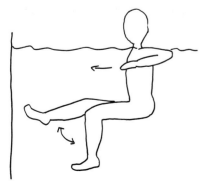

Fig. 9.9: Breast stroke arms cossack legs

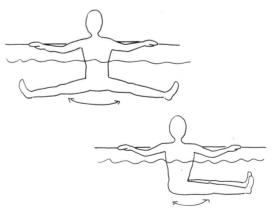

Fig. 9.13: Back braced scissors

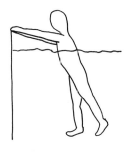

Fig. 9.14: Front lean flat-footed backward kicks (alternate feet 15 cm (6") off pool floor)

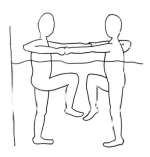

Fig. 9.15: Washerwoman jog

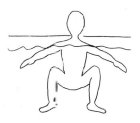

Fig. 9.16: Tuck jumps

Guidelines for Running Aquafitness Classes

The following are general guidelines for running Aquafitness classes:

1. Don't enter or leave the water abruptly. This can cause rapid changes in blood pressure which may be dangerous in some people.

2. Don't exercise with the head under water or while holding the breath.

3. Where possible ensure there is protection if the bottom of the pool is slippery. Old sand shoes with holes cut in them to let the water out can be useful.

4. Avoid exercises involving excessive extension of the lower back, particularly while using the pool-side for support.

5. Avoid using over-heated pools (over 30 degrees C) for general exercise classes, as they can cause a build-up of heat in the body (stretch and movement classes, however, may be carried out in temperatures up to 33 degrees C).

6. Warm up and cool down gradually, as in all exercise classes. When starting, include exercises to increase circulation to the lower legs and feet.

7. Ensure that all participants can swim or are sufficiently confident, at least, in water. Inability to swim should not exclude a person from participating, but instructors ought to be aware of individuals' limitations.

8. Don't forget that showering and using skin moisturiser and anti-fungal power on the feet is recommended after water classes.

9. Close attention should be paid to participants at all times to ensure that no one is getting cold, tired or in any way distressed.

10. Instructors should be aware of the environment in which they are working, e.g., who is responsible for providing emergency services, where the telephone is located, etc., and have a detailed knowledge of cardio-pulmonary resuscitation, water rescue techniques and first aid.

10 Fitness Testing

It is vital to assess an individual's physical fitness before prescribing an exercise program. Fitness assessments of one kind or another are used for the following reasons:

1. To cater for the needs of an individual and monitor his/her progress.
2. To diagnose or verify heart disease and the extent of damage; also to measure improvement during subsequent therapeutic programs.
3. To screen for athletic abilities and detect weak spots for improvement.

In this chapter, only a basic testing protocol will be considered. This is meant for the fitness centre and not for the sophisticated testing laboratory. Detailed tests and those involving cardiac function should only be carried out under the strict supervision of a suitably qualified person.

When selecting fitness tests for assessing new members or re-assessment of current members the following should be borne in mind:

• Select tests that are suitable to a cross section of the population
• Select tests that are non-threatening
• Select tests that are informative to the tester and also to the person being tested
• Select tests that are motivational
• Select tests that have comparison tables
• Select tests that are repeatable
• Select tests that do not require technical or medical supervision.

Fitness Testing for the Fitness Centre

The following tests have been selected specifically for instructors who wish to find out about the general health and fitness of a client while making the experience as non-threatening as possible.

1. Life-style screening questionnaire

2. Blood pressure
3. Resting heart rate
4. Height and weight — Static tests
5. Skinfold measures
6. Girth measures

7. Stamina (aerobic):
  • Bicycle ergometer test
    or
  • Step-up test
8. Suppleness (flexibility): — Dynamic tests
  • Sit and reach
9. Strength (endurance):
  • Crunch test
10. Life-style counselling

Pre-Test Screening

Fitness testing is a form of physical examination. It usually involves physical activity and hence the question often asked is, 'can it be dangerous?'

Says the famous Swedish exercise physiologist Per Olaf Astrand: 'The question is frequently raised whether a medical examination is advisable before commencing a training program. Certainly anyone who is doubtful about his state of health should consult a physician. In principle, however, there is less risk in activity than in continuous inactivity. *In a nutshell, our opinion is that it is more advisable to pass a careful medical examination if one intends to be sedentary in order to establish whether one's state of health is good enough to stand the inactivity.*'

For those under 35 years of age, with no obvious health risk (e.g. high blood pressure, a history of heart disease, overweight, diabetes mellitus), a fitness test serves as motivation, to check on progress at a later stage. For others, it might be useful as a screening device, and to help devise a program to suit special needs.

Figure 10.1 is a simple screening test for determining the need for a medical clearance prior to being prescribed an exercise program.

	Score
Age:	
under 35	0
35–44	1
45–54	2
55 & over	4
Obesity level:	
Normal weight	0
More than 20% overweight	2
Blood pressure:	
under 140/90	0
under 160/95	2
over 160/95	4
not known	2
Medical history:	
previous cardiac trouble	6
diabetes mellitus	5
heart disease in family	2
heavy smoking (> 10 day)	2
previously inactive	1
pregnancy	5
lower back pain	5

Fig. 10.1: Sample Pre-test Screening Questionnaire

Anyone scoring 5 or more points on the scale should be comprehensively screened by a suitably qualified person before beginning exercise. Those scoring under 5 can begin a graded exercise program without comprehensive testing.

The **Exercise Safety Questionnaire** developed by Jamie Hayes, managing director of Aerobic City in Sydney, is an excellent example of how a fitness centre has adapted a comprehensive lifestyle screening questionnaire to the specific needs of the fitness industry (Figure 10.2). The relevant lifestyle questions have been summarised into eight sentences and the client is only asked to give a yes or no to each question. If the client answers *yes* or *not sure* to any question then the instructor discusses the matter further and either recommends that the client gets a medical clearance or, as will often be the case, the client will be given a light exercise program to commence with.

The remaining questions asked in the Aerobic City lifestyle screen give the management an indication of whether their advertising is working and what are the fitness goals of potential members.

Techniques of Fitness Assessment

There are numerous methods available for assessing the various components of physical fitness. Some are elaborate and time-consuming and require sophisticated equipment, but many others are both simple and reliable. If proper procedures are followed they can provide information for a total fitness profile such as that shown in Table 10.15 at the end of this chapter.

The tests considered here in detail will cover the

EXERCISE SAFETY QUESTIONNAIRE

FOR YOUR SAFETY
please answer the following questions by ticking the appropriate box and read the EXERCISE
ADVICE below ....

tick to answer ☑

		NO	YES or not sure
1.	Have you ever had any injury, illness, back or joint condition that may be aggravated by vigorous exercise?	☐	☐ ☞
2.	Have you ever had: Arthritis, Asthma, Diabetes, Epilepsy, Hernia, dizziness, Gout, circulation problems or an Ulcer?	☐	☐ ☞
3.	Have you ever had a Heart condition, High Blood Pressure, Rheumatic Fever, Stroke, High Cholesterol, palpitations, murmers or pains in the chest?	☐	☐ ☞
4.	Have your mother, father, brother or sister had any heart problems prior to age 60?	☐	☐ ☞
5.	Are you now or have recently been pregnant?	☐	☐ ☞
6.	Are you taking any prescribed medication?	☐	☐ ☞
7.	Is there any other condition that might be reason to modify your exercise programme?	☐	☐ ☞
8.	Have you been doing regular vigorous exercise lately?		
	If YES, what type of exercise?		

> PLEASE CHECK WITH YOUR DOCTOR OR SPECIALIST BEFORE EXERCISING

EXERCISE ADVICE

BEGINNERS   Start by attending the circuit classes. Work at a slow pace and learn how to do each exercise correctly. On each visit you will be able to work a little harder. Please ask the circuit class instructor for guidance.

REGULARS   Regular exercisers can attend either the circuit classes or the floor classes. Take your time learning any new exercises. Please wear proper Aerobics shoes in all floor classes.

PLEASE   Start at a sensible pace as you are responsible for the health of you own body. Should your health status change in the future please tell us.

Name:... .

Address: ....P'Code: ....

Work Phone: .... Employer: ....

How would you describe your current physical condition?
☐ Unwell   ☐ Overweight   ☐ Unfit   ☐ "Healthy"   ☐ Fit

What are the main benefits that you want from exercise?
☐ Fat loss   ☐ Improve Fitness   ☐ Increase size   ☐ Social enjoyment
☐ Muscle tone   ☐ Maintain Fitness   ☐ Sport training   ☐ Good health

To improve you fitness, exercise at least 3 time per week. Fitness assessments are recommended to help you start safely and to monitor you progress. For advice or assistance just ask any staff.

How did you find out about Aerobic City? ....

I have completed the EXERCISE SAFETY QUESTIONNAIRE and understand the EXERCISE ADVICE above.

Signed _____ Date_____   © Aerobic City 1988

T: .... C/C: .... I: .... E: .... S: ....
SU: .... B: .... M: .... C: ....

Fig. 10.2: Aerobic City Exercise Safety Questionnaire

areas of anthropometry (body measurements), blood pressure, cardiovascular endurance, flexibility, and muscular strength and endurance.

Other more specific tests (agility, power, speed etc.)

can be obtained from more detailed testing manuals (see reference section).

Table 10.1 shows some common tests used in the areas to be considered here.

Table 10.1: Some common tests for evaluating physical fitness

Fitness components	Tests	Comments
Cardiorespiratory endurance (VO_2 max)	Treadmill	Coupled with gas analyses, is the best test available.
	Bicycle ergometer	Simple yet accurate and safe.
	Bench stepping	Simple in design and operation
	12 minute run	Field test with minimal facility.
Muscular strength	Sit-ups	Measures abdominal strength.
	Dynamometer	Measures handgrip strength, back lift and leg lift strength.
	Tensiometer	Measures strength of 38 muscle groups.
	Weight lifting	Measures body strength and power
Muscular endurance	Chin-ups	Measures arm and shoulder endurance
	Flexed arm hang	Measures forearm, biceps, and upper back muscle endurance.
	Pull-ups	Measures arm and shoulder endurance
	Push-ups	Measures pectoral muscle endurance
	Sit-ups	Measures abdominal endurance.
Flexibility	Sit and reach test	Measures static flexibility at the hip joint
	Bend, twist and touch test	Measures trunk flexibility
	Leighton's flexometer	Measures flexibility of all joints in degrees.

Anthropometry

The main anthropometric measures of value to the fitness leader are height and weight and body fat. Height/weight ratios are also often used as a combined measure of obesity or overweight (i.e. the Ponderal or Quetelet indices). However, because these indices don't take into account the extent of lean body mass (LBM) and bony structure, they are usually inappropriate as a measure of fatness.

Body weight is also an inappropriate measure of the effectiveness of a fitness program. As a result of training, an individual can lose fat but gain LBM or muscle. Because muscle is heavier than fat, total body weight may *increase* rather than decrease in the early

stages of training. There may also be an increase in glycogen storage in body muscle with training. As glycogen attracts fluid (approximately 2.7 grams of water to each gram of glycogen), this can also mean an increase in body weight in the early stages of training.

A more accurate guide to overfatness is the direct measurement of body fat. The standard measure for this is underwater weighing. Because fat floats and lean muscle tends to sink, a direct measure can be made between the difference in body weight when measured out of water and of body weight estimated from the displacement of water when the body is submerged.

Measuring Body Fat

In most clinical or applied situations, underwater weighing is impractical. The next best approximation is the assessment of fat using skin-fold measurements taken with special skinfold calipers.

The skinfold caliper should have a pressure of 10 gm/mm² irrespective of the design of the caliper. A useful size of the contact surface lies in the neighbourhood of 20 to 40 mm², and depends in part on the shape of the contact surface. The skin should be lifted by grasping firmly a fold between the thumb and forefinger at about a distance of 1 cm from the site at which the skinfold is to be measured.

General Guide and Comments

Taking accurate and repeatable skinfold measurements depends on accurate location of the site of measurement, forming the skinfold prior to the application of the caliper jaws, the standardisation of the alignment of the skinfold crest, and the complete release of the spring handles of the caliper so that the full standard pressure of the jaws is applied to the soft tissues being measured.

The pointer on the dial of the skinfold caliper should be allowed to steady and the drift to cease before measurements are recorded. Precise measuring and marking of the level of the skinfold are necessary because subcutaneous fat thickness varies substantially over the areas being measured.

Although skinfold measurements are generally simple to carry out, the correct procedure requires much practice. Tester error is the most common source of variation in measurements.

Common Sites Used

1. *Skinfold over triceps:* Located on the dorsum of the right upper arm (over the triceps), at the marked level halfway between the acromial process (collar-bone) and olecranon process (elbow). In measuring this skinfold, the arms should hang freely. The crest of the skinfold is parallel to the long axis of the upper arm.

2. *Skinfold over biceps:* Located on the ventral side of the upper arm (over the biceps), at the marked level halfway between acromion and olecranon. The crest of the skinfold is parallel to the long axis of the upper arm.

3. *Subscapular skinfold:* Located about 1 cm below the lower angle of the right scapula with the subject standing in a relaxed position. The crest of the skinfold is medially upward and laterally downward at about 45 degrees.

4. *Suprailiac skinfold:* Located about 3 cm above the suprailiac crest (hip bone). The crest of the skinfold is vertical.

British researchers Durnin and Womersley measured skinfold thickness at the above 4 sites and calibrated these with underwater weighing, deriving the equivalent fat content as a percentage of body weight. From this they developed tables of body fat norms by age (see Table 10.2).

Procedure

1. Pick up the skinfold between the thumb and forefinger about 1 cm above the skin-marks, with the crest of the fold following the alignment specified, and apply the caliper jaws to the exact site.

2. Release the spring handles fully.

3. When the pointer of the dial has steadied, read off the measurements in tenths of millimetres.

4. Take 3 readings for each site and average the 3 readings.

Estimation of Leanness and Fatness

Using Table 10.2, the sum of these four skinfolds can be converted to percent body fat. For example, if a sum total of the four skinfold thicknesses amounts to

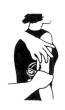 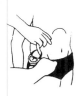 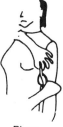 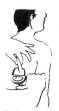

Triceps   Suprailiac   Bicep   Subscapular

Fig. 10.3: Common skinfold sites

Table 10.2: Percent body fat by age (Durnin and Womersley, 1974)

Males (age in years)				
Sum of skinfolds (mm)	17–19	20–29	30–39	40–49	50+

Sum of skinfolds (mm)	17–19	20–29	30–39	40–49	50+
15	5.00	4.64	9.09	8.47	8.38
16	5.75	5.58	9.74	9.31	9.31
17	6.44	6.08	10.35	10.09	10.19
18	7.10	6.74	10.93	10.84	11.02
19	7.72	7.37	11.48	11.54	11.80
20	8.32	7.96	12.00	12.22	12.55
21	8.89	8.53	12.50	12.86	13.27
22	9.43	9.07	12.97	13.47	13.95
23	9.95	9.59	13.43	14.06	14.60
24	10.45	10.09	13.87	14.62	15.23
25	10.92	10.57	14.29	15.16	15.84
26	11.39	11.03	14.69	15.68	16.42
27	11.83	11.48	15.08	16.19	16.98
28	12.26	11.91	15.46	16.67	17.53
29	12.67	12.32	15.82	17.14	18.05
30	13.07	12.73	16.17	17.60	18.56
31	13.46	13.12	16.51	18.04	19.05
32	13.84	13.49	16.84	18.47	19.53
33	14.21	13.86	17.16	18.88	19.99
34	14.56	14.22	17.47	19.28	20.44
35	14.91	14.56	17.77	19.68	20.88
36	15.25	14.90	18.07	20.06	21.31
37	15.57	15.23	18.36	20.43	21.73
38	15.89	15.55	18.63	20.79	22.13
39	16.21	15.86	18.91	21.15	22.53
40	16.51	16.17	19.17	21.49	22.92
41	16.81	16.47	19.43	21.83	23.29
42	17.10	16.76	19.69	22.16	23.66
43	17.38	17.04	19.93	22.48	24.02
44	17.66	17.32	20.18	22.80	24.38
45	17.93	17.59	20.41	23.11	24.72
46	18.20	17.86	20.65	23.41	25.06
47	18.46	18.12	20.87	23.71	25.39
48	18.71	18.37	21.10	24.00	25.72
49	18.96	18.63	21.31	24.28	26.04
50	19.21	18.87	21.53	24.56	26.35
51	19.45	19.11	21.74	24.83	26.66
52	19.69	19.35	21.95	25.10	26.96
53	19.92	19.58	22.15	25.37	27.26
54	20.15	19.81	22.35	25.63	27.55
55	20.37	20.04	22.54	25.88	27.83
56	20.59	20.26	22.73	26.13	28.11
57	20.81	20.47	22.92	26.38	28.39
58	21.02	20.69	23.11	26.62	28.66
59	21.23	20.90	23.29	26.86	28.93
60	21.44	21.11	23.47	27.09	29.20
61	21.64	21.31	23.65	27.33	29.45
62	21.84	21.51	23.82	27.55	29.71
63	22.04	21.71	23.99	27.78	29.96
64	22.23	21.90	24.16	28.00	30.21
65	22.42	22.09	24.33	28.22	30.45
66	22.61	22.28	24.49	28.43	30.70
67	22.80	22.47	24.66	28.64	30.93
68	22.98	22.65	24.81	28.85	31.17
69	23.16	22.83	24.97	29.06	31.40
70	23.34	23.01	25.13	29.26	31.63

Sum of skinfolds (mm)	17–19	20–29	30–39	40–49	50+
71	23.52	23.19	25.28	29.46	31.85
72	23.69	23.36	25.43	29.66	32.07
73	23.86	23.53	25.58	29.85	32.29
74	24.03	23.70	25.73	30.04	32.51
75	24.20	23.87	25.87	30.23	32.72
76	24.36	24.03	26.01	30.42	32.93
77	24.52	24.20	26.16	30.61	33.14
78	24.68	24.36	26.30	30.79	33.35
79	24.84	24.52	26.43	30.97	33.55
80	25.00	24.67	26.57	31.15	33.75
81	25.15	24.83	26.70	31.33	33.95
82	25.31	24.98	26.84	31.50	34.15
83	25.46	25.13	26.97	31.67	34.34
84	25.61	25.28	27.10	31.85	34.53
85	25.76	25.43	27.23	32.01	34.72
86	25.90	25.58	27.36	32.18	34.91
87	26.05	25.72	27.48	32.35	35.10
88	26.19	25.87	27.61	32.51	35.28
89	26.33	26.01	27.73	32.67	35.46
90	26.47	26.15	27.85	32.83	35.64
91	26.61	26.29	27.97	32.99	35.82
92	26.75	26.42	28.09	33.15	36.00
93	26.89	26.56	28.21	33.30	36.17
94	27.02	26.70	28.32	33.45	36.35
95	27.15	26.83	28.44	33.61	36.52
96	27.28	26.96	28.55	33.76	36.69
97	27.42	27.09	28.67	33.91	36.85
98	27.54	27.22	28.78	34.05	37.02
99	27.67	27.35	28.89	34.20	37.19
100	27.80	27.48	29.00	34.34	37.35
101	27.92	27.60	29.11	34.49	37.51
102	28.05	27.73	29.22	34.63	37.67
103	28.17	27.85	29.33	34.77	37.83
104	28.29	27.97	29.43	34.91	37.99
105	28.42	28.09	29.54	35.05	38.14
106	28.54	28.21	29.64	35.19	38.30
107	28.65	28.33	29.74	35.32	38.45
108	28.77	28.45	29.85	35.46	38.60
109	28.89	28.57	29.95	35.59	38.75
110	29.00	28.68	30.05	35.72	38.90
111	29.12	28.80	30.15	35.85	39.05
112	29.23	28.91	30.25	35.98	39.20
113	29.35	29.03	30.34	36.11	39.34
114	29.46	29.14	30.44	36.24	39.48
115	29.57	29.25	30.54	36.37	39.63
116	29.68	29.36	30.63	36.49	39.77
117	29.79	29.47	30.73	36.62	39.91
118	29.90	29.58	30.82	36.74	40.05
119	30.00	29.69	30.91	36.86	40.19
120	30.11	29.79	31.01	36.99	40.33
121	30.22	29.90	31.10	37.11	40.46
122	30.32	30.00	31.19	37.23	40.60
123	30.43	30.11	31.28	37.35	40.73
124	30.53	30.21	31.37	37.46	40.87
125	30.63	30.31	31.46	37.58	41.00

Females				
15	10.40	10.22	13.50	16.40	17.85
16	11.21	11.08	14.27	17.15	18.65
17	11.98	11.89	14.99	17.87	19.40

Sum of skinfolds (mm)	17–19	20–29	30–39	40–49	50+
18	12.71	12.66	15.68	18.54	20.11
19	13.40	13.39	16.33	19.18	20.79
20	14.05	14.08	16.95	19.78	21.44
21	14.68	14.75	17.54	20.36	22.05
22	15.28	15.38	18.10	20.92	22.64
23	15.85	15.99	18.64	21.45	23.20
24	16.40	16.57	19.16	21.96	23.74
25	16.93	17.13	19.66	22.44	24.26
26	17.44	17.67	20.14	22.91	24.76
27	17.93	18.19	20.60	23.37	25.24
28	18.40	18.69	21.05	23.80	25.71
29	18.86	19.17	21.48	24.23	26.16
30	19.30	19.64	21.90	24.64	26.59
31	19.73	20.10	22.31	25.03	27.01
32	20.15	20.54	22.70	25.42	27.42
33	20.56	20.97	23.08	25.79	27.82
34	20.95	21.39	23.45	26.16	28.21
35	21.33	21.79	23.81	26.51	28.58
36	21.71	22.19	24.16	26.85	28.95
37	22.07	22.57	24.51	27.19	29.30
38	22.42	22.95	24.84	27.51	29.65
39	22.77	23.31	25.16	27.83	29.99
40	23.10	23.67	25.48	28.14	30.32
41	23.43	24.02	25.79	28.45	30.64
42	23.76	24.36	26.09	28.74	30.96
43	24.07	24.69	26.39	29.03	31.26
44	24.38	25.02	26.68	29.32	31.57
45	24.68	25.34	26.96	29.59	31.86
46	24.97	25.65	27.24	29.87	32.15
47	25.26	25.96	27.51	30.13	32.43
48	25.54	26.26	27.78	30.39	32.71
49	25.82	26.55	28.04	30.65	32.98
50	26.09	26.84	28.30	30.90	33.25
51	26.36	27.12	28.55	31.14	33.51
52	26.62	27.40	28.79	31.39	33.77
53	26.88	27.68	29.04	31.62	34.02
54	27.13	27.94	29.27	31.86	34.27
55	27.38	28.21	29.51	32.09	34.51
56	27.63	28.47	29.74	32.31	34.75
57	27.87	28.72	29.96	32.53	34.99
58	28.10	28.97	30.19	32.75	35.22
59	28.34	29.22	30.40	32.96	35.45
60	28.57	29.46	30.62	33.17	35.67
61	28.79	29.70	30.83	33.38	35.89
62	29.01	29.94	31.04	33.58	36.11
63	29.23	30.17	31.25	33.79	36.32
64	29.45	30.40	31.45	33.98	36.53
65	29.66	30.62	31.65	34.18	36.74
66	29.87	30.84	31.84	34.37	36.95
67	30.07	31.06	32.04	34.56	37.15
68	30.28	31.28	32.23	34.74	37.35
69	30.48	31.49	32.32	34.93	37.54
70	30.67	31.70	32.60	35.11	37.74
71	30.87	31.91	32.79	35.29	37.93
72	31.06	32.11	32.97	35.47	38.12
73	31.25	32.32	33.14	35.64	38.30
74	31.44	32.51	33.32	35.82	38.49
75	31.62	32.71	33.49	35.99	38.67
76	31.81	32.91	33.67	36.15	38.85
77	31.99	33.10	33.84	36.32	39.02

Sum of skinfolds (mm)	17–19	20–29	30–39	40–49	50+
78	32.17	33.29	34.00	36.48	39.20
79	32.34	33.47	34.17	36.65	29.37
80	32.52	33.66	34.33	36.81	39.54
81	32.69	33.84	34.49	36.96	39.71
82	32.86	34.02	34.65	37.12	39.88
83	33.03	34.20	34.81	37.28	40.04
84	33.19	34.38	34.97	37.43	40.20
85	33.36	34.55	35.12	37.58	40.36
86	33.52	34.73	35.28	37.73	40.52
87	33.68	34.90	35.43	37.88	40.68
88	33.84	35.07	35.58	38.02	40.84
89	34.00	35.23	35.72	38.17	40.99
90	34.15	35.40	35.87	38.31	41.14
91	34.31	35.56	36.01	38.45	41.29
92	34.46	35.72	36.16	38.59	41.44
93	34.61	35.88	36.30	38.73	41.59
94	34.76	36.04	36.44	38.87	41.74
95	34.91	36.20	36.58	39.00	41.88
96	35.06	36.36	36.72	39.14	42.03
97	35.20	36.51	36.85	39.27	42.17
98	35.34	36.66	36.99	39.40	42.31
99	35.49	36.82	37.12	39.53	42.45
100	35.63	36.97	37.25	39.66	42.59
101	35.77	37.11	37.38	39.79	42.72
102	35.91	37.26	37.51	39.92	42.86
103	36.04	37.41	37.64	40.04	42.99
104	36.18	37.55	37.77	40.17	43.13
105	36.31	37.69	37.90	40.29	43.26
106	36.45	37.84	38.02	40.41	43.39
107	36.58	37.98	38.15	40.54	43.52
108	36.71	38.12	38.27	40.66	43.65
109	36.84	38.25	38.39	40.77	43.77
110	36.97	38.39	38.51	40.89	43.90
111	37.10	38.53	38.63	41.01	44.02
112	37.22	38.66	38.75	41.13	44.15
113	37.35	38.80	38.87	41.24	44.27
114	37.47	38.93	38.98	41.36	44.39
115	37.60	39.06	39.10	41.47	44.51
116	37.72	39.19	39.21	41.58	44.63
117	37.84	39.32	39.33	41.69	44.75
118	37.96	39.45	39.44	41.80	44.87
119	38.08	39.57	39.55	41.91	44.99
120	38.20	39.70	39.66	42.02	45.10
121	38.32	39.83	39.78	42.13	45.22
122	38.43	39.95	39.88	42.24	45.33
123	38.55	40.07	39.99	42.34	45.45
124	38.66	40.20	40.10	42.45	45.56
125	38.78	40.32	40.21	42.55	45.67

Table 10.3: Classification of leanness and fatness based on percent fat for general population

	Men	Women
Lean	<12.0%	<17.0%
Acceptable	12.0–20.9%	17.0–27.9%
Mod. overweight	21.0–25.9%	28.0–32.9%
Overweight	≥26.0%	≥33.0%

Table 10.4: Classification of leanness and fatness for male and female athletes based on percent body fat

	Male athletes	Female athletes
Lean	<7.0%	<12.0%
Acceptable	7.0–14.9%	12.0–24.9%
Overweight	≥15.0%	≥25.0%

74 mm, then using Table 10.2 for men or for women, one could read across the table on the column with the appropriate age-group. For a man aged 35 years with a skinfold thickness of 74 mm, his percent body fat is 25.73. This means that 25.7% of his body weight is made up of fat tissue, i.e. 18.0 kg of adipose tissue is present in his body if his body weight is 70.0 kg. The corresponding value for a woman is 33.32% or 20.0 kg of fat in a body weighing 60.0 kg.

The average fat content for a young, healthy adult man is 10–15% and for a young, healthy adult woman is 18–25%. The average older men and women have 5 to 10% more fat than their younger counterparts.

However, the increase in body fat content with age is not necessarily physiologically desirable or healthy. Classification of leanness and fatness based on percent body fat is necessarily arbitrary. Nevertheless, Table 10.3 gives an arbitrary classification for the general population.

Body fat content is obviously affected by physical activity. There is a wide variation in body fat content ranging from 4 to 20% for male athletes, and 10 to 26% for female athletes. Certainly the types of sporting activity and the amount of physical training involved are important determinants of body composition in elite athletes. Again, classification of leanness and fatness for average athletes is necessarily arbitrary. Table 10.4 serves as a guide for such a classification.

When taking skinfold measures and counselling people on their percent body fat levels, instructors should be sensitive to the feelings of the client. Terms such as 'moderately obese' and 'body fat' should be replaced with 'higher than is generally accepted' and 'extra weight'.

Blood Pressure

Blood pressure is the measure of the force the heart needs to push blood through the body. A simple definition of blood pressure is: 'The resistance of the blood against the artery walls'.

A good analogy, when explaining blood pressure, is the force of water in a hose pipe. If the hose is thin or blocked in any way, the same force of water at the tap will cause a higher pressure against the walls of the hose. If, on the other hand, the hose has a large opening and the water is free flowing, the pressure of the water against the hose will be low. The same is true for the arterial blood vessels. If there is too much pressure on the artery walls this places additional strain on the heart.

There are two different measures of blood pressure:

i) The *systolic measure* which is the contraction phase of the heart or the pumping pressure of the heart
ii) The *diastolic measure* which is the relaxation phase of the heart or the pressure in the arteries when the heart is filling up with blood.

These two measures are expressed as systolic over diastolic and an acceptable range is considered to be:

Systolic 120 ± 10
Diastolic 80 ± 10

Recording Blood Pressure

Blood pressures can be measured by the auscultatory method, using a sphygmomanometer and a stethoscope. A sphygmomanometer consists of a cuff, a mercury manometer (or anaroid manometer), and an inflating bulb with exhaust control (see Figure 10.3). The stethoscope is used to listen to the sounds of blood flow. The cuff is wrapped around the arm. When the brachial artery is occluded by increasing the cuff pressure 30 mm Hg above the expected systolic pressure, there is no blood flowing to the forearm and no sound is heard through the stethoscope. As the cuff pressure is lowered slowly to a point at which systolic blood pressure just exceeds the cuff pressure, a tapping sound can be heard. The cuff pressure at which the first sound is heard is called the *systolic blood pressure*. As the cuff pressure is lowered further, the sound becomes louder, then dull and muffled, and finally disappears. These are the 'sounds of Korotkow'. The abrupt muffling of the arterial sound signals that blood flow is no longer impeded by the cuff pressure, and this is the *diastolic blood pressure*. Blood pressures are usually expressed in millimetres of mercury (mm Hg).

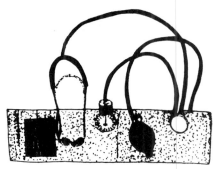

Fig. 10.4: A common sphygmomanometer for measuring blood pressure

Blood pressures vary considerably throughout the day and night, according to a variety of conditions. Posture, breathing, emotion, exercise, cigarette smoking and caffeine can cause a rise or fall in blood pressure. If a subject has not engaged in physical activity for 2 hours prior to testing, has not been under emotional stress, has not been smoking or drinking caffeinated beverages for the previous 2 hours and has been seated comfortably for half an hour prior to blood pressure recording, variations can be minimised and false diagnoses can be avoided.

The World Health Organisation has defined a systolic blood pressure of more than 160 mm Hg and a diastolic blood pressure of more than 95 mm Hg as abnormal and requiring treatment and continuous observation. Blood pressure consistently below 140 mm Hg for systolic and 90 mm Hg for diastolic can be regarded as being normal.

The National Heart Foundation states that a person who records a blood pressure measure of 140/90 has borderline hypertension (high blood pressure) and further medical examination is recommended. This is especially so if the person wishes to participate in an exercise program.

Instructors are reminded that anyone can take blood pressure, but diagnosis and counselling of hypertension should be done only by appropriately medically qualified people.

Procedure

1. Sit the subject with arm outstretched. Loosen the control valve on the cuff of the 'sphygmo' by turning it anti-clockwise so that air is released entirely from the cuff.

2. Wrap the cuff around the subject's arm, with the lower edge 2 cm above the crease at the elbow. Ensure that the stethoscope on the cuff is against the skin.

3. Close the control valve and pump the bulb to raise the cuff pressure to a level of about 160–180 mm Hg on the manometer.

4. Gradually open the control valve so that the needle slowly moves downward as the cuff pressure is released. The rate of pressure drop should be 2–3 mm Hg per second.

5. The first sound heard through the stethoscope indicates the pressure at which blood again begins to flow to the forearm. This is taken as the *systolic blood pressure*.

6. Allow the cuff pressure to continue to fall. Note that the sound becomes louder, then dull and muffled, and disappears altogether. The point at which the sound becomes muffled is the *diastolic blood pressure*.

7. Deflate the cuff entirely. Allow for 1–2 minutes rest and repeat the above procedure to obtain a second reading.

Evaluating Cardiorespiratory Endurance (Stamina)

Cardiorespiratory endurance can be measured in a number of ways, the standard being the direct measurement of oxygen uptake. This requires sophisticated equipment to measure expired respiratory gases while the subject is exercising at a maximal level. Measurements can be carried out on a treadmill, exercise bicycle, rowing machine or similar aerobic exercise machine.

For practicality, the maximum (or 'max') test is not always appropriate and hence a number of sub-maximal tests can be used. In these cases, the subject is exercised to a pre-set level (not exhaustion), and extrapolations are made from norm tables to estimate maximal oxygen uptake (VO_2 max).

Submaximal aerobic tests estimate maximal oxygen uptake (VO_2 max) based on heart rate following a set workload. This estimate is based on the physiological principle that there is a direct and linear relationship between heart rate and workload (see Figure 10.5).

As aerobic fitness improves there is a reduction in heart rate for the same workload (see Figure 10.5). This is the basis of all submaximal tests that use heart rate

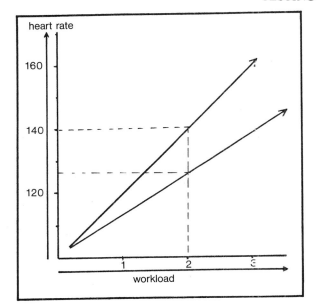

Figure 10.5: Relationship between heart rate and workload

as a measure of intensity. It should be noted however, that the heart rate and workload relationships are only valid at a certain heart rate range and are not linear at very high or very low heart rates. Thus, given a certain workload, and the heart rate measured at the steady state of work, the maximum oxygen uptake can be predicted with a known degree of accuracy.

The advantages and disadvantages of the most common submaximal tests are summarised in Table 10.5 over page.

A Sub-Maximal Test Using the Bicycle Ergometer

Although VO₂ max is primarily dependent on the cardiorespiratory function of man, it is also dependent on the duration and nature of the task, the mass of muscle involved, fatigue levels, and environmental conditions such as climate and altitude.

The bicycle ergometer is perhaps the most adaptable instrument in the laboratory for aerobic testing. It is simple to use, cheap, occupies little space and is easily transportable. It's also sufficiently versatile to provide a number of different work loads.

Work on the bicycle ergometer is calculated in kilopondmetres/minute. A *kilopondmetre* (kpm) is the amount of force required to move a mass of 1 kg through a distance of 1 metre. A *watt* (which is also often used as a measure of work) equals 6.12 kpm/min.

Before being tested on the bicycle ergometer, a subject should satisfy the following:

Pre-testing Conditions

1. No meal should be taken for 1–2 hours prior to the test.
2. No vigorous exercise for at least 24 hours.
3. No smoking for 1 hour.
4. No caffeinated drinks (tea, coffee, cola) for at least 1 hour.
5. Subjects on blood pressure medication should consult their doctor about refraining from medication for 24 hours prior to testing, if possible.

Testing Procedure

The following is the testing procedure for an Astrand/Ryhming sub-maximal bicycle test.

1. Testing should be carried out in an environment of around 20 degrees C.
2. Ensure the subject is comfortable on the bike. Saddle height should allow for completely stretched leg at the lowest pedal point.
3. Practise taking resting pulse while the subject is seated. This can be done at either the neck (carotid pulse) or wrist (radial pulse). If a heart rate meter or electrocardiograph (ECG) is used, these should be regularly calibrated.
4. Determine a workload suitable for the subject.
5. After commencing exercise, ensure that the subject is pedalling at a steady pace at the desired workload. While pedalling, the subject should remain seated.
6. After 1 minute of exercise, a satisfactory heart rate would be 116–128 bpm. An underload or overload would be noticed at 1–2 minutes and appropriate adjustments made to the work load.
7. The ideal heart rate of steady state of exercise is 120–170 beats per minute (depending on age).
8. Measure heart rate for 15 seconds every minute on the minute and multiply this by 4 to get HR per minute. This should be done for 7 minutes and scores recorded on a data sheet.
9. Average the 5th and 6th minutes of heart rate if there was no alteration of work load since the start of exercise; otherwise average the 6th and 7th minutes of heart rates. Enter this average heart rate as the work heart rate.
10. Record the workload at this point on the data sheet.
11. If the subject experiences discomfort while exercising, the test should be stopped immediately.

Table 10.5: Advantages and disadvantages of common sub-maximal VO₂ max tests.

Test	Time required	Procedure	Advantages	Disadvantages	Estimated relation with VO₂ max test
12–15 min. run	12–15 mins	Distance covered; formulae for determining VO₂ for trained and untrained athletes	Simplicity; no equipment	• Needs learning for pacing • Favours runners/walkers • High stress level	85–90%
Astrand Bicycle ergometer	6 mins	Constant workload on cycle ergometer, VO₂ max estimated from tables of heart rate (HR). HR taken between 5–6th minute	Time; simplicity; reasonably accurate; appropriate for ECG monitoring	• Variability in Max HR in individuals • favours cyclists • underestimates for those with a high maximum HR • As max HR decreases with age, the test over-estimates fitness with advancing age. Correction factors must be used	89–90%
PWC₁₇₀	9 mins	3 workloads on cycle ergometer at 3 min. intervals. By graphing HR responses to these workloads, work which can be completed at a HR of 170 can be estimated	Clear steps on protocol; gradual increase in work intensity; reasonably accurate; appropriate for ECG monitoring	• time involved in graphing results • difficulty in gauging 170 bpm level accurately • favours cyclists	89–90%
Harvard Step Test	3–5 mins +3 mins measuring	Step at rate of 30 steps/min on 45.5 cm step. HR recorded at 1½, 2½ and 3½ mins. after stopping	Minimal equipment; easy to conduct; can be self administering	• high stress level • inappropriate for children • influenced by variations in max HR	60–80%
Queen's College Step Test	3 mins + 15 secs. measuring	Step at rate of 24 steps/min (men), 22 steps/min (women) on 42.5 cm step. HR recorded for 15 secs, 5 secs after stopping.	Minimal equipment; easy to conduct; little time required; can be self administering	• influenced by variations in max HR	60–80%

Calculation of VO₂ max

Using the working heart rate and the exercise load, VO₂ max can be calculated from the tables provided for men and women (Tables 10.6 and 10.7).

As maximum heart rate decreases with age, a correction factor for age is needed. This can be done by multiplying the maximum oxygen uptake with the correction factor for the appropriate age range (see Table 10.8).

The figures provided by the following tables are in litres per minute. This can be converted to millilitres per minute by multiplying by 1000. A measure for VO₂ max can then be determined by dividing by body weight (in kilograms).

Example of a VO₂ max calculation

Age: 35 years
Sex: Male
Body weight: 72.0 kg
Workload: 900 kpm/min

Heart rate: 147 bpm
Predicted VO₂ max: 3.3 litres/min (Table 10.6)
Age correction factor: 3.3 l/min × 0.87 = 2.871 l/min (Table 10.8)
VO₂ max expressed on a weight basis: 2.871 × 1000/72.0 = 39.8 ml/kg/min
Comparison tables: Average VO₂ max for age (Table 10.9)

Standards for VO₂ max

Australian standards for maximum oxygen uptake are scarce although tables have been developed from work carried out by the Human Performance Laboratory at the Sydney College of Advanced Education. Table 10.9 gives fitness levels for men and women aged 20–59. Table 10.10 gives comparative figures for Australian boys and girls.

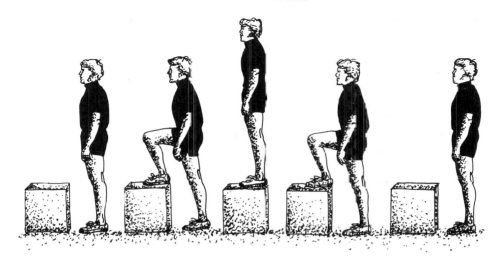

Fig. 10.6: Measuring aerobic fitness using the step test

The Step Test

A less accurate but more convenient sub-maximal measure of aerobic capacity for the fitness centre is the step test. There are a number of different step test measures with the two most common being the Harvard Step Test and the Queen's College Step Test.

i) The Harvard Step Test

The Harvard Step Test is based on *heart rate recovery* following a given work load. This consists of 3 or 5 minutes of stepping up and down on an 18 inch step, followed by pulse measurements at 1½, 2½ and 3½ minutes after finishing stepping.

ii) The Queen's College Step Test

The Queen's College is a simpler step test developed by Professor William McArdle. This test is based on *heart rate following* a given workload, not recovery heart rate as is the case with the Harvard Step Test.

Testing Procedure for the Queen's College Step Test

1. Obtain a 16 inch step. This can be easily constructed or simply use a solid chair.

2. Have a cadence tape or metronome to ensure the correct stepping speed.

3. Have the subject start with both feet on the floor and facing the step. Practice the stepping cycle as follows:

- up—right foot up
- up—left foot up
- down—right foot down
- down—left foot down

Ensure that when on the box or chair both legs are straight (see Figure 10.6).

4. Once the subject has started stepping he or she must keep in time with the cadence. For women this should be 22 stepping cycles per minute and for men 24 stepping cycles.

5. The subject must maintain the stepping cycle for three minutes. However, after 1½ minutes the subject changes the leg he or she started stepping up on. This prevents too much overload on one leg.

6. Throughout the test the instructor should regularly monitor how the subject is feeling. If the subject feels any discomfort the test should be stopped and the heart rate and duration of the test recorded.

7. Immediately following 3 minutes of stepping the subject should stop stepping and be asked to sit on the stepping box or chair. Within five seconds the instructor should begin counting heart rate for 15 seconds. Multiply this by 4 to give the heart rate per minute.

8. Compare the result with the scores from Table 10.11.

Estimates have also been made of VO$_2$ max from step tests, but it should be emphasised that like all sub-maximal tests, these are subject to error.

Table 10.6: Prediction of maximum oxygen uptake from heart rate and work load on a bicycle ergometer

MALES

	Maximum Oxygen Uptake Litres/min.				
Heart Rate	300 kpm/min.	600 kpm/min.	900 kpm/min.	1200 kpm/min.	1500 kpm/min.
120	2.2	3.5	4.8		
121	2.2	3.4	4.7		
122	2.2	3.4	4.6		
123	2.1	3.4	4.6		
124	2.1	3.3	4.5	6.0	
125	2.0	3.2	4.4	5.9	
126	2.0	3.2	4.4	5.8	
127	2.0	3.1	4.3	5.7	
128	2.0	3.1	4.2	5.6	
129	1.9	3.0	4.2	5.6	
130	1.9	3.0	4.1	5.5	
131	1.9	2.9	4.0	5.4	
132	1.8	2.9	4.0	5.3	
133	1.8	2.8	3.9	5.3	
134	1.8	2.8	3.9	5.2	
135	1.7	2.8	3.8	5.1	
136	1.7	2.7	3.8	5.0	
137	1.7	2.7	3.7	5.0	
138	1.6	2.7	3.7	4.9	
139	1.6	2.6	3.6	4.8	
140	1.6	2.6	3.6	4.8	6.0
141		2.6	3.5	4.7	5.9
142		2.5	3.5	4.6	5.8
143		2.5	3.4	4.6	5.7
144		2.5	3.4	4.5	5.7
145		2.4	3.4	4.5	5.6
146		2.4	3.3	4.4	5.6
147		2.4	3.3	4.4	5.5
148		2.4	3.2	4.3	5.4
149		2.3	3.2	4.3	5.4
150		2.3	3.2	4.2	5.3
151		2.3	3.1	4.2	5.2
152		2.3	3.1	4.1	5.2
153		2.2	3.0	4.1	5.1
154		2.2	3.0	4.0	5.1
155		2.2	3.0	4.0	5.0
156		2.2	2.9	4.0	5.0
157		2.1	2.9	3.9	4.9
158		2.1	2.9	3.9	4.9
159		2.1	2.8	3.8	4.8
160		2.1	2.8	3.8	4.8
161		2.0	2.8	3.7	4.7
162		2.0	2.8	3.7	4.6
163		2.0	2.8	3.7	4.6
164		2.0	2.7	3.6	4.5
165		2.0	2.7	3.6	4.5
166		1.9	2.7	3.6	4.5
167		1.9	2.6	3.5	4.4
168		1.9	2.6	3.5	4.4
169		1.9	2.6	3.5	4.3
170		1.8	2.6	3.4	4.3

Table 10.7: Prediction of maximum oxygen uptake from heart rate and work load on a bicycle ergometer

FEMALES

	Maximum Oxygen Uptake Litres/min.				
Heart Rate	300 kpm/min.	450 kpm/min.	600 kpm/min.	750 kpm/min.	900 kpm/min.
120	2.6	3.4	4.1	4.8	
121	2.5	3.3	4.0	4.8	
122	2.5	3.2	3.9	4.7	
123	2.4	3.1	3.9	4.6	
124	2.4	3.1	3.8	4.5	
125	2.3	3.0	3.7	4.4	
126	2.3	3.0	3.6	4.3	
127	2.2	2.9	3.5	4.2	
128	2.2	2.8	3.5	4.2	4.8
129	2.2	2.8	3.4	4.1	4.8
130	2.1	2.7	3.4	4.0	4.7
131	2.1	2.7	3.4	4.0	4.6
132	2.0	2.7	3.3	3.9	4.5
133	2.0	2.6	3.2	3.8	4.4
134	2.0	2.6	3.2	3.8	4.4
135	2.0	2.6	3.1	3.7	4.3
136	1.9	2.5	3.1	3.6	4.2
137	1.9	2.5	3.0	3.6	4.2
138	1.8	2.4	3.0	3.5	4.1
139	1.8	2.4	2.9	3.5	4.0
140	1.8	2.4	2.8	3.4	4.0
141	1.8	2.3	2.8	3.4	3.9
142	1.7	2.3	2.8	3.3	3.9
143	1.7	2.2	2.7	3.3	3.8
144	1.7	2.2	2.7	3.2	3.8
145	1.6	2.2	2.7	3.2	3.7
146	1.6	2.2	2.6	3.2	3.7
147	1.6	2.1	2.6	3.1	3.6
148	1.6	2.1	2.6	3.1	3.6
149		2.1	2.6	3.0	3.5
150		2.0	2.5	3.0	3.5
151		2.0	2.5	3.0	3.4
152		2.0	2.5	2.9	3.4
153		2.0	2.4	2.9	3.3
154		2.0	2.4	2.8	3.3
155		1.9	2.4	2.8	3.2
156		1.9	2.3	2.8	3.2
157		1.9	2.3	2.7	3.2
158		1.8	2.3	2.7	3.1
159		1.8	2.2	2.7	3.1
160		1.8	2.2	2.6	3.0
161		1.8	2.2	2.6	3.0
162		1.8	2.2	2.6	3.0
163		1.7	2.2	2.6	2.9
164		1.7	2.1	2.5	2.9
165		1.7	2.1	2.5	2.9
166		1.7	2.1	2.5	2.8
167		1.6	2.1	2.4	2.8
168		1.6	2.0	2.4	2.8
169		1.6	2.0	2.4	2.8
170		1.6	2.0	2.4	2.7

Table 10.8: Correction factors

Age	Factor	Maximum Heart Rate	Factor
15	1.10	210	1.12
25	1.00	200	1.00
35	0.87	190	0.93
40	0.83	180	0.83
45	0.78	170	0.75
50	0.75	160	0.69
55	0.71	150	0.64
60	0.68		
65	0.65		

These factors are to be used for correction of estimated maximum oxygen uptake. 1. for age differences, or 2. when the subject's maximum heart rate is known.

Table 10.9: Maximum oxygen uptake (ml. kg. $^{-1}$ min $^{-1}$ STPD) for Australians.

	Men			
Age	**20–29**	**30–39**	**40–49**	**50–59**
Poor	Less than 41.9	Less than 35.3	Less than 30.8	Less than 29.4
Fair	42.0–46.3	35.4–38.9	30.9–34.4	29.5–32.8
Average	46.4–51.0	39.0–42.6	34.5–39.2	32.9–36.0
Good	51.1–55.0	42.7–49.9	39.3–44.7	36.1–40.3
Excellent	55.1 or more	50.0 or more	44.8 or more	40.4 or more
	Women			
Age	**20–29**	**30–39**	**40–49**	**50–59**
Poor	Less than 30.0	Less than 26.0	Less than 23.9	Less than 21.0
Fair	30.1–34.9	26.1–29.9	24.0–27.9	21.1–23.9
Average	35.0–39.9	30.0–33.0	28.0–30.9	24.0–28.9
Good	40.0–45.0	33.1–40.9	31.0–37.9	29.0–34.9
Excellent	45.1 or more	41.0 or more	38.0 or more	35.0 or more

Table 10.10: Maximum oxygen uptake (ml. kg. $^{-1}$ min $^{-1}$ STPD) for Australian boys and girls.

		Boys			
Age	**Poor**	**Fair**	**Average**	**Good**	**Excellent**
12	≤46.0	46.1–47.8	47.9–51.5	51.6–53.3	53.4+
13	≤46.0	46.1–47.8	47.9–51.5	51.6–53.3	53.4+
14	≤46.1	46.2–49.7	49.8–53.4	53.5–55.2	55.3+
15	≤44.8	44.9–48.4	48.5–52.1	52.2–55.7	55.8+
16	≤40.0	40.1–44.8	44.9–49.7	49.8–54.5	54.6+
17	≤34.3	34.4–40.3	40.4–46.4	46.5–52.4	52.5+

		Girls			
Age	**Poor**	**Fair**	**Average**	**Good**	**Excellent**
10	≤36.4	36.5–42.4	42.5–48.5	48.6–54.5	54.6+
11	≤36.4	36.5–42.4	42.5–48.5	48.6–54.5	54.6+
12	≤36.7	36.8–40.7	40.8–44.8	44.9–48.8	48.9+
13	≤34.2	34.3–37.8	37.9–41.5	41.6–45.1	45.2+
14	≤33.5	33.6–37.5	37.6–41.6	41.7–45.6	45.7+
15	≤30.1	30.2–34.5	34.6–39.0	39.1–43.4	43.5+
16	≤33.4	33.5–37.0	37.1–40.7	40.8–44.3	44.4+

Table 10.11: Step test scores

| | Exercise Pulse | | | |
Rating	Men	Women	Boys	Girls
Very good	<110	<116	<120	<124
Good	100–124	116–130	120–130	124–134
OK	125–140	131–146	131–150	135–154
Poor	141–155	147–160	151–160	155–164
Very poor	>155	>160	>160	>165

Evaluating Flexibility

Flexibility is the ability to move part or parts of the body in a wide range of movement without undue strain to the articulations and muscle attachments. Since the degree of flexibility in various joints of the same individual may differ greatly, it is considered specific to the joint involved. By the proper use of standard instruments and tests it is possible to determine which individuals (and which joints of the body) have the greatest flexibility.

For many sports, flexibility is all-important. In the normal person, graceful movement in walking and running is dependent on a certain amount of flexibility. It is also believed that maintaining good joint mobility can prevent or relieve the aches and pains that grow more common with age.

Static flexibility measures the range of movement. It does not measure the stiffness or looseness of the same joint during movement.

Dynamic flexibility refers to the ease of movement of joints in the middle of their range of movement.

The Sit-and-Reach Test (Static Flexibility)

The sit-and-reach test is measured with a simple piece of equipment (see Figure 10.7). If this is not available, a ruler can be placed between the legs with the measure starting at the soles of the feet and moving away from the body.

Procedure
1. This measure should be taken following a total body warm-up. It is best carried out following an aerobic sub-max test.

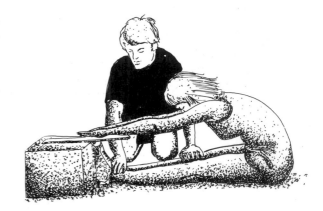

Fig. 10.7: Measuring trunk flexion

2. The subject sits on the floor with feet on either side of the ruler and pressed against the front board (see Figure 10.7).
3. Keeping the knees straight, the subject bends at the trunk and gradually pushes the indicator as far forward as possible.
4. Three readings should be taken and the best measure recorded. These can be compared with figures in Table 10.12 below.

Table 10.12: Flexibility classification

| | Static Flexibility (cm) | |
Age	20–39	40–59
Poor	≤1.0	≤−6.0
Fair	1.1–6.0	−5.9–1.0
Average	6.1–10.0	1.1–7.0
Good	10.1–13.0	7.1–10.0
Excellent	13.1+	10.1+

Evaluating Muscular Strength and Endurance

Strength is defined as the ability to carry out work against a resistance. The amount of muscular force which can be exerted against a resistance depends on the size and number of muscles involved; the proportion of muscle fibres engaged in the action; the co-ordination of the muscle groups; the physical condition of the muscle groups; and the mechanical advantage of the bones employed.

A variety of different techniques are used to measure strength, two of the most convenient being the grip dynamometer test of handgrip strength and the crunch test for abdominal strength and endurance.

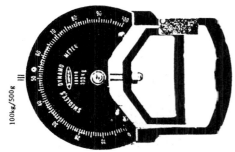

Fig. 10.8: Smedley's Handgrip Dynamometer

Procedure for Measuring Handgrip Strength

1. The subject holds the dynamometer in one hand, in line with the forearm and hanging by the thigh.
2. The dynamometer is gripped between the fingers and palm at the base of the thumb.
3. When firmly grasped, it is held away from the body and squeezed vigorously, the subject exerting the maximum force of which he/she is capable.
4. The arm should not be swung or pumped violently. This may increase the recorded score.
5. 2 trials should be allowed for each hand, each score being noted. Only the better result counts. Compare with Table 10.13 below.

Table 10.13: Classification of Handgrip Strength

	Men		Women	
	Left	Right	Left	Right
Excellent	68	70	37	41
Very good	56	62	34	38
Above average	52	56	30	33
Average	46	50	25	29
Below average	43	48	22	25
Poor	41	45	19	23
Very poor	39	41	18	22

Endurance, like strength, can be specific to a particular muscle group. Hence muscular endurance can be measured by a variety of techniques stressing different muscles. One common and relevant measure is that of abdominal muscle endurance which can be gauged through the 20, 30, 60 or 120 second crunch test.

Procedure for Measuring Abdominal Strength and Endurance

1. The subject lies on the floor with feet on a standard-height chair so the knees are bent at right angles.
2. Fold the arms in front of the chest with elbows pointing forward.
3. The subject raises the shoulders off the ground in a 'crunch' position until the elbows touch the thighs. Return then to the position of shoulders flat on the ground

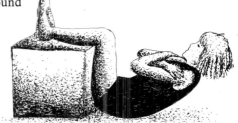

Fig. 10.9: Measuring abdominal strength

4. Practice should be allowed first.
5. Have the subject carry out as many complete crunches as possible in 20 seconds. If the elbows do not touch the thighs, or the shoulders are not returned to the flat-on-the-ground position, the crunch isn't counted.
6. Score the number of crunches completed in either 20, 30, 60 or 120 seconds. Norms for 20 seconds are shown in Table 10.14.

Table 10.14: Abdominal strength measure

Strength rating	Sit-ups completed		
	Age		
	<29	30–39	40–59
Good	>17	>15	>13
OK	12–17	11–15	10–13
Poor	<12	<11	<10

The Fitness Profile

From the tests above, a complete fitness profile can be developed (see Table 10.15). This enables the tester to design a program to meet specific needs as well as providing ready information for the subject to evaluate improvements in fitness at some later point.

Table 10.15: The Fitness Profile

The Fitness Profile Chart

Name: _____

Membership No. _____ Lifestyle screen: _____ Test date: _____

Test measures	Score	Rating
Blood pressure: i) Systolic measure ii) Diastolic measure		
Body fat – skinfold sites: i) Triceps _____ ii) Biceps _____ iii) Sub-scapular _____ iv) Supra-iliac _____ Total		

	Score	Rating

Stamina fitness
  (aerobic)
i)   Step test
      or
ii) Bike test		

Suppleness test
  (flexibility)
  Sit and reach		

Strength test i) Grip strength ii) Crunch test (endurance)		

Lifestyle counselling

i)   Comments: _____

ii)   Recommendations: _____

Guidelines for Exercise Testing

1. Any instructor carrying out sub-maximal testing must be trained by personnel qualified in the protocol being used.

2. Tests used must be standardised (preferably with local norm tables). If other tests are devised, these should have readily accessible figures for validity and reliability.

3. All tests must be carried out to rigid specifications. Attention should be paid in particular to small aspects such as straightening of the knees on a step test, or relaxing a client before a blood pressure measurement.

4. All equipment used in testing must be standard and regularly calibrated to the manufacturer's standards.

5. If telemetric devices such as EEGs, ECGs or EMGs are used for monitoring, the personnel using such equipment must be fully trained in their use.

6. Maximal testing must be carried out to a strictly observed protocol. Oxy-viva equipment must be available. Personnel carrying out the testing must be fully qualified and this should only be carried out

where access to emergency medical services can be made within 5 minutes.

7. All testing must be preceded by a pre-test screen (preferably a written questionnaire). Clients not fulfilling the standards set by this screen (e.g. National Heart Foundation Guidelines or see Figure 10.1) should then not be tested unless under the supervision of a qualified exercise physiologist or medical practitioner.

8. All testing must be clearly monitored by qualified personnel.

9. Testing must cease at the client's request.

10. Testing should always be followed by a detailed counselling session advising the client of results and, where appropriate, prescribing an individual exercise program to suit the needs of that client.

11. If a battery of tests is used, these must be so ordered sequentially as to not influence the outcome of each test. For example, blood pressure should be taken *before* sub-maximal testing and *after* a brief quiet period, such as completing the screening questionnaire.

12. Where norms are used, these must be based on a large heterogeneous population and must be up to date and preferably (although not always) of local origin.

13. Unless specifically aiming to measure one aspect of fitness (e.g. aerobic capacity), testing should involve at least tests of flexibility, aerobic fitness and body composition. Each type of testing should be carried out to protocols laid down in standard texts or journal publications.

14. Body weight/body fat measures must include an assessment of skinfold thickness as well as overall weight. The relevance of this should be explained to the client in any subsequent counselling session, and the use of body weight as a measure of fatness should be de-emphasised.

15. Where a test is intended as a means of medical diagnosis, a medical practitioner must be involved before information is transmitted to the client.

16. Clients must be given written information about pre-test requirements such as not eating or not drinking caffeinated drinks before testing. Clients should also be questioned about their immediate exercise efforts to determine whether the effects of any test may be affected by a recent heavy workload.

17. If blood is drawn this should be by a qualified person with suitably clean provisions applying. Blood should be analysed by a scientifically acceptable laboratory.

18. Adequate warm-up and cool-down procedures must apply for all clients participating in testing. These should have in mind the specific test to be carried out. For example, flexibility testing should be preceded by stretching to avoid injury to 'cold' muscles and joints.

19. All tests must be specific to the purpose. Thus if increased strength or endurance is an aim of a follow-up program, tests for these should be included.

11 Weight Control and Exercise

About 50% of middle aged Australians and 25% of young Australians are overweight (that is, carrying more than 25% body mass as fat). Data on school children over time indicate that this proportion has increased over the past 30–40 years, despite the fact that the average Australian now consumes no more than his or her grandparents. The difference appears to be in the amount of energy burned up, i.e. exercise.

In the past, use of a certain amount of energy was a necessary part of daily life; walking, farming, chopping wood, bicycling etc. However, with the advent of modern technology, particularly the motor car, the engine and energy saving devices such as lifts and escalators, daily energy use has declined. When coupled with no decline in food intake, the result is an excess of fat.

The Dangers of Excess Fat

The reason most people want to lose weight is to improve appearance. Modern society doesn't look kindly on extra poundage, and millions of dollars each year are spent in trying to remove it.

In earlier times, when only the wealthy could over-eat and remain sedentary, a corpulent figure was regarded as a sign of affluence. Now, with food abundant, the opposite is usually more true. Still the medical disadvantages of being overweight remain.

By being overweight, an individual puts himself or herself at increased risk of illnesses such as hypertension (high blood pressure), heart disease, stroke, diabetes and gallstones. In addition, he or she can generally expect a shorter lifespan, with added risks during pregnancy, childbirth and surgery and an aggravation of existing medical conditions like arthritis. There are also the very real effects of loneliness, rejection, lack of self-esteem and lack of energy.

Overweight and Obesity

It's been known for a long time that body weight is influenced by the balance between food energy taken in and exercise energy expended; the formula being:

Energy balance = Energy in − energy out.

The equivalent amounts of exercise regarded as necessary to balance various food intakes are shown in Table 11.1. Remember that 1 kg of body fat is equivalent to about 32,500 kJ (7600 kcals) of energy. According to this analysis, food intake in excess of

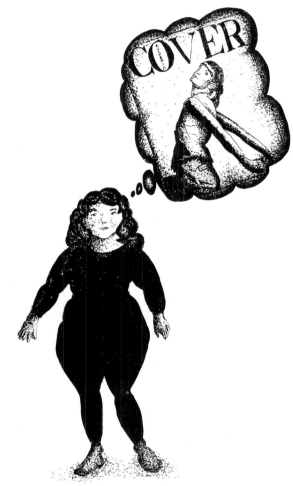

Fig. 11.1: Effective weight control means not setting unrealistic goals

of individual factors. It's obvious, for example, that some people put on more weight than others with a given level of food intake and it's thought that this may have something to do with the ability of some bodies to use up energy more efficiently than others.

Heredity and family upbringing also play a part. Studies indicate that two parents of normal weight have only a 7% chance of having overweight children, whereas if one parent is fat, there is a 40% chance that the children will be overweight, and if both parents are fat, there is an 80% chance.

Body weight is thought to be a function of two processes: hypertrophy and hyperplasia of body fat cells. *Hypertrophy* is the enlargement of existing fat cells which occurs either through inactivity or excessive food intake. It is perhaps the most common form of weight increase. *Hyperplasia* on the other hand is an increase in fat cell numbers, which also results in an increase in body weight and size. Hyperplasia was typically not thought to be responsible for most body weight increases, because fat cell numbers were thought to be laid down early in life and to be relatively incapable of change. Recent research suggests that fat cell numbers may be significantly changed through eating and exercise habits at 3 particular stages in life. These are:

1. Before birth, i.e. during foetal development
2. In the early years (between 1–2) of life
3. In early adolescence (i.e. 12–14 years).

Once cell numbers are increased it is thought that they cannot be reduced at a later point, except in size (atrophy). Hence, lifestyle factors are seen as vital at these stages for developing a body structure which will aid in weight control.

Research has also concentrated recently on a homeostatic mechanism within each individual which may control that person's possible upper and lower weight limits. Yet, although many ideas have been put forward to explain the possible imbalance between

daily energy needs leads to obesity which is, basically, an excess of fat.

And while the energy formula remains roundly true, recent research has begun to highlight the importance

Table 11.1: Caloric Intake of Foods and Caloric Expenditure of Selected Activities

Type of food	Calories per serving	Kilojoules	Minutes required for expenditure					
			Sleeping	Bowling	Golf	Walking	Tennis	Jogging
Large apple	101	424	87	23	20	20	14	10
Boiled egg	77	323	66	17	15	15	11	7
Bread and butter	78	328	67	18	16	16	11	7
Two strips bacon	96	403	82	22	19	19	14	9
Glass beer	114	479	98	26	23	23	16	10
Glass milk	166	697	142	38	33	32	33	15
Cheese pizza	180	756	154	41	36	35	25	16
T-bone steak	235	987	201	53	47	45	33	23
Hamburger	350	1470	300	80	70	67	49	32
Strawberry shortcake	400	1680	343	91	80	77	56	37

energy intake and energy output, as yet no unifying theory has emerged. All we can say is that *people are different*. Hence, while certain reduction methods might be effective and easy for some, they may not work for others.

Exercise, Diet and Weight Control

For many, weight control means dieting. There's a general belief that only small amounts of energy are burned up during quite extensive exercise and that therefore calorie restriction is more effective than exercise in influencing the energy balance formula.

Scientific research has done little to modify this view. In fact, despite wide interest in weight control, there are few acceptable scientific studies supporting the use of exercise in weight control programs.

Those that have been reported are often poorly conceived, badly controlled or inadequately interpreted. Yet an examination of the physiological data shows the following:

1. Exercise doesn't necessarily increase the appetite, as many people think. Studies with both animals and humans indicate that with a moderate increase in exercise intensity there is a *decrease* in appetite and food intake. World authority on weight control, Professor Jean Mayer of Harvard University, puts this down to the fact that *lack of* exercise in the sedentary person causes an increase in food intake which is only corrected by returning the body to its 'normal' level of exercise. At high energy usage rates, e.g. athletes, heavy physical workers etc, food intake can increase by up to 300% (see Table 11.2). However, because of the high energy output, these people still do not put on weight.

2. Exercise increases the *basal metabolic rate (BMR)*, or the rate at which the body uses energy at rest to sustain vital bodily functions. Studies carried out have

shown that the BMR may remain at least 10% above the resting state for up to 48 hours after exercise, hence higher energy use continues during this period.

3. The post-exercise elevation of BMR has been estimated to be responsible for up to 3 kg of body fat loss over a year following regular (i.e. 20 minutes a day, 3–4 times a week), mild exercise.

Table 11.2: Daily Energy Intake of Competitive Sportspeople

Sport	Average body weight, kilograms	Estimated daily cal intake
Cross-country skiing	67.5	6105
Bicycle racing	68.0	5995
Canoe racing	75.0	5995
Marathon racing	68.0	5940
Soccer	74.0	5885
Field hockey (men)	75.0	5720
Handball (European)	75.0	5610
Basketball	75.0	5610
Ice hockey	68.0	5390
Gymnastics (men)	67.0	5000
Sailing	74.0	5170
Fencing	73.0	5000
Sprinting (track)	69.0	4675
Boxing (middle and welter weight)	63.5	4675
Diving	61.0	4620
Pole vault	73.0	4620

(From *Encyclopaedia of Sport Sciences and Medicine* by the American College of Sports Medicine)

The Energy Costs of Dieting

The energy needs of an individual are based on that person's exercise or activity requirements and on the *basal metabolic rate* (BMR). The BMR is defined as the energy needs of the body at complete rest in a fasting state, i.e. it is the amount of energy necessary to sustain life.

BMR is influenced by a number of factors including:

1. *Body size and composition:* Tall thin people with a larger body surface area to weight ratio experience greater heat loss than short muscular individuals, hence

their BMR is higher. However, when the temperature of the environment is greater than that of the body (i.e. 37.5 degrees C), the situation is reversed due to the greater surface area of the thin person which increases the absorption of heat by convection. Because muscle is approximately twice as dense as fat, a muscular person will also have a higher BMR than a person of equivalent body weight with a higher fat content.

2. *Age:* BMR tends to decrease with age. It is greatest during periods of rapid growth in childhood, and during the growth spurt associated with puberty. BMR declines in adulthood at the rate of about 2% per decade. If diet and exercise remain constant, the individual will gain weight as he/she gets older.

3. *Sleep:* Sleep can lower BMR by 10–15%, hence the amount of sleep an individual gets may be relevant.

4. *Environmental conditions:* Climatic conditions can affect BMR such that individuals in tropical areas may exhibit BMRs as much as 10–20% lower than when they are in temperate climates.

5. *Sex:* Because females in general have a 5–10% higher fat content than males (and because fat is less dense than muscle), BMRs in females are often lower than those in males. Other factors, such as hormones may also play a role in the sex differences in BMR.

Ironically, BMR is generally reduced during dieting because of a thermic effect (i.e. the actual energy cost of digesting food), which may be up to 10% of the caloric intake. Some studies also show that dieting can cause a significant decrease in the energy costs of exercise of anything up to 25%. The end result seems to be a plateauing of weight loss from dieting, which may only be reduced by the increased metabolic rate of exercise.

From a comprehensive review of the literature on obesity and exercise carried out in 1982, Professor Kevin Thompson from the University of Georgia concludes that:

'Researchers have extensively used caloric restriction as an intervention even though the body's adaptive lowering of expenditure during food deprivation is an established fact of energy balance. The rejection of exercise as a valid treatment has resulted from a narrow focus on its immediate role in energy expenditure to the exclusion of other relevant metabolic and physiological changes that accompany training.'

This view has led some researchers to question the value of dieting in weight loss. At the extremes it has been suggested that 'dieting can make you fat'. This, it is proposed, may occur because dieting leads to losses in lean body mass (LBM), as well as fat. But LBM (which is basically muscle), is heavier and therefore is thought to use more energy (BMR) than fat. Hence BMR may decrease during dieting, meaning that when the diet ceases and the person returns to regular eating, fat may be put on more easily.

In reality, the best solution to weight control lies in a balanced exercise and food intake program. It is true that fad and crash diets don't work because much of the losses are fluids, which are soon replaced. It's also true that exercise has been vastly under-rated in many weight loss programs.

However, an effective program of weight control must be something that can be maintained as a lifestyle habit. Hence a balance between the appropriate exercise techniques and proper diet is likely to be most effective.

Problems with Exercise as a Means of Weight Loss

While exercise is perhaps an underrated form of weight control, it should be recognised that it is not without its problems. In the first place, many people who need to lose weight are extremely unfit. At this level they may find it difficult to achieve a sufficient level of activity to lose much weight.

For the obese, the most comfortable forms of activity are those that are weight supportive, e.g. swimming, cycling. And while these can be good aerobic forms of exercise, they need to be carried out at a sufficient intensity and duration to develop a training effect. They also assume a certain skill level—a poor swimmer, for example, is unlikely to be able to swim at an aerobic rate for a long enough period to achieve the desired effects.

For this reason a combination of exercise and diet is desirable in the early stages of a weight reduction program. This combined approach will achieve weight loss without the reduction in lean muscle mass that would occur with diet alone. It should be recognised, however, that tiredness while exercising may be more common with this approach. Also, because there may be increases in muscle size and stores of glycogen (which stores water), there may be increases rather than decreases in body weight in the early stages, even though body dimensions may decrease because of losses of fat.

General Principles of Weight Control

To be effective, any weight control program should do the following:

1. **Involve changes that can be maintained for life:** Crash dieting followed by a return to gluttony cannot help maintain slimness.

2. **Have gradual, long-term and realistic goals:** A gradual loss of 0.5 kg per week is realistic without being masochistic.

3. **Utilise both dietary and exercise changes:** Cutting back on food by 1000 kJs a day can lead to an 11 kg weight loss in a year. But walking an extra 3 kilometres a day can double that.

4. **Incorporate a nutritionally balanced diet:** Many fad diets don't have the essential elements necessary for a healthy diet.

5. **Take account of the real causes of obesity:** Blaming over-eating for obesity is akin to blaming beer for alcoholism. A successful weight reduction program will operate on the *cause* and not the *effect* of over-eating.

Dieting: the Good and the Bad

Exercise as a weight control technique has been covered throughout this manual. But as we've pointed out, the best forms of weight control incorporate exercise and food restriction. The latter can take many forms.

There are literally hundreds of diets available including 'water diets', 'fat or protein diets', 'drinking man's diets' and many other 'fad diets'. In many cases these involve sheer quackery, like notions that water before a meal will 'dilute' the calories consumed, or that foods such as grapefruit can alter the calorific value of other foods. In other cases, such as high fat and low carbohydrate diets, the dangers aren't as obvious, but many medical organisations advise strongly against them.

While there may even be big initial weight losses with some fad or gimmicky diets, these generally involve fluid loss which is quickly replaced. In general, provided a diet is nutritionally balanced, it doesn't matter what's eaten, but how many kilojoules it contains. Diets that do not involve kilojoule reduction (either obviously or unobviously) are unlikely to work on a long-term basis.

Within this restriction there are several effective diet types which cater for the different characteristics of the person dieting. Two effective diet type plans are *pre-planned diets* and *self-directed diets*.

Pre-Planned Diets

For people who prefer to be directed in their dieting, pre-planned diets provide one answer. Meals are pre-planned and divergences from them are not allowed.

This type of program requires the ability of the dieter to have control over his/her meals. Those faced with business lunches, travelling or regular entertainment may find it difficult to maintain. It should also be pointed out that spartan diets like the Pritikin regime need a commitment to long-term lifestyle change if they are to work properly.

Self-Directed Diets

Self-directed diets are those that offer alternative foods or reduced portions rather than a strict meal plan. They therefore provide more variety than planned diets. But they also require more of the dieter.

Self-directed diets are best for individuals who do not like to be strictly directed by an outside source. They require a good knowledge of the calorie contents of various foods and confidence in one's own level of self-control.

Self-directed diets are rarely glamorous or gimmicky, but in the long run they are likely to be the most effective. Recommended Australian plans include those put out by State and Federal Government Departments (*Your Health and Your Figure*, Commonwealth Govt Printer, 1980; *Losing Weight Wisely*, Health Dept of NSW, 1980; and others (e.g. Borushek, A: *The Complete Diet Manual for Australian Weight Watchers*, 1978).

The Psychology of Eating

Eating can be a habit. In advanced Western countries, eating is probably less influenced by hunger than the cues that have come to be associated with food. For example, we learn to eat 3 meals at set times of the day, whether we're really hungry or not.

Like a rat that learns to press a bar for food in response to a light, or Pavlov's dogs that learned to salivate at the sound of a bell, people become conditioned to the cues that are associated with eating.

In one study carried out some time ago, overweight and normal weight people were placed in an enclosed room with access to food. A clock on the wall was their only clue to the time of day. For one group of subjects the clock was slightly speeded up, while for the others it remained at normal speed.

Overweight people in the experiment tended to eat more from the ad-lib food supply when the clock time (irrespective of the real time) approached normal meal time. Normal weight people were less influenced by the clock.

This suggests that the cues associated with eating are perhaps stronger for some people than others. In these cases the chances of over-eating are obviously greater, and these people are perhaps more likely to be overweight. Simply reducing food intake, then, while it may be an admirable goal, may not be enough in a weight control program; a more comprehensive technique will involve principles of behaviour modification.

Modification of Eating Behaviour

Reducing food intake can involve a major modification of learned behaviour and often lifestyle in general. Psychological techniques of behaviour modification therefore offer promise for long-term and permanent change. These can be learned through either group (e.g. Weight Watchers), or self-management techniques.

The first step in eating-behaviour modification is to identify the various eating characteristics of the individual, i.e. records should be kept for some time before dieting is even begun. These records should include the following:

1. What is eaten when and where (e.g. in front of TV, at work, in the kitchen).
2. The feelings of the dieter at the time (e.g. depressed, anxious, excited).
3. How much time was spent eating?
4. Other associated cues (seated at a table, eating from the refrigerator, etc.).
5. What activities were carried out while eating (talking, socialising, watching TV)?
6. Who was present during the meal?

A careful analysis of these records can provide the dieter with clues about the eating habit. The next step is to try and break down the conditioned effect by breaking these signals to eat. One way is to substitute alternative behaviour, e.g instead of eating while driving, sing along with the radio; instead of eating while watching TV, paint, write or draw; instead of eating when depressed, do 10 minutes of pre-defined exercise; instead of eating while relaxing, have no food in relaxation areas.

Other useful techniques are restricting eating to 1 location, making eating a ritual that can't be carried out at irregular intervals, using smaller portions of food, eating slowly, chewing frequently for each mouthful, using reward techniques for success.

An overweight person has generally taken years to become so. Changes in learned behaviour won't occur overnight. However, without an effort to modify the behaviours—both exercise and nutrition—that have contributed to the problem in the first place, there's little prospect of a lifelong solution. A guide to the individual variables hypothesised to be involved in the variety of weight control techniques discussed in this chapter is shown in Figure 11.2.

	Self Management			Dieting	
	Exercise plans	Individual	Group	Self directed	Pre planned
If you like direction			X		X
If you like company			X		
If you have strong self-control	X	X		X	
If you don't like going hungry	X			X	
If you are prepared to change your lifestyle significantly					X
If you don't mind paying to lose weight		X	X		
If you are the meticulous type		X		X	

Fig. 11.2: A Guide to Reduction Programs

Spot Reduction

'Spot' reduction or the loss of weight from specific areas of the body, is sometimes promised by certain 'health' institutions. However, research has shown convincingly that spot reduction does *not* occur. Fat is burned from *all* body stores as a result of exercise, rather than just the region of muscle being exercised.

One study, reported in an unpublished thesis at Illinois University, looked at the effects of mild isometric, isotonic, strength and flexibility exercises on fat specific to the upper arm, waist, hips and thighs of a group of women.

The exercises were carried out over 30 minutes a day, 3 days a week for 10 weeks. Results were compared with a control group who did no organised exercise during that time. Exercises used included some which are commonly used in spot reduction programs, e.g. sit-ups, trunk twists, arm circles, side-lying leg raises, back bicycle, hip walk, windmills and leg extensions.

The results showed that there were no differences between controls and the exercising group on girth measures or body weight at the end of the exercise period. This suggests that not only did 'spot reduction' not occur, but that the exercises were probably too mild even for any significant aerobic effect.

Other research shows that even when a dominant arm is used during exercise, skinfold fat decreases in both arms at the same rate. Also, when intensity of exercise is equated through heart rate measures, generalised aerobic exercise is as effective as specific spot exercises in spot reducing.

In the normal person it appears that fat is lost from fat stores over the entire body as a result of energy use. Hence any form of aerobic exercise will be as effective in reducing a bulging waistline as any stomach exercise. In most cases aerobic exercise will be even more effective because it can be carried out at a greater rate of continuous energy usage.

Cellulite

Cellulite is the term given (for no apparent reason) to the quilted cottage cheese-like fat effect found on the neck, breasts, arms and particularly thighs of some people—generally women. The term was invented in the 1930s, and in fact has no medical usage.

Despite varied claims of cure, there is little known about the nature of cellulite except that it's a form of fat. The term describes a condition of fatty tissue which is resistant to the normal stimuli for fat breakdown.

It is assumed that cellulite differs in structure and metabolism from other fatty tissue, but the differences are not fully understood. Proposed causes are circulation problems and the effects of female hormones, particularly in cases where obesity does not seem to play a role. Again these causes are not proven.

Fat is removed from the body in areas of excess in response to energy utilising activity. It does *not* respond to spot reduction programs aimed at exercising only the part of the body at which fat deposits are present. The best known technique for its removal is aerobic exercise coupled with a sensible reduction in total energy intake, particularly fat, sugar and alcohol.

There is no form of passive exercise—rubs, baths, oils, brushes—that is effective in the long-term removal of cellulite. Reductions of salt in the diet may help because of the fluid-retaining effect of this substance.

Guidelines for Weight Control Programs

The following guidelines should be considered in any comprehensive weight control program:

1. Programs involving diet should ensure that all dietary advice is based on sound, nutritionally balanced information.

2. There should be no use of 'passive exercise' devices for weight loss purposes where there is no sound experimental evidence for supporting the use of such equipment. Ineffective devices include figure-wrapping creams, sauna suits, sauna pants, electric stimulators and vibrating belts and rollers.

3. All diets should be structured for long-term, gradual weight loss rather than quick, large losses.

4. Fad diets that are not nutritionally balanced or supported by scientific research should not be used at any time.

5. Short-term goals as well as long-term goals should be set; these should be concentrated on an average weekly loss of 0.5–1 kg.

6. There is a difficulty in using body weight as a measure of improvement because of differences in body shape. Where possible, skinfold thickness and girth measurements should be used.

7. Records should be kept to monitor effort and progress over time.

8. There should be some analysis of eating behaviour in dietary management and some attempts made to incorporate modification of such behaviour in any weight control program.

9. Where weight gain is indicated through increased food intake, this should be through an increase in a balanced mix of food rather than through 'empty' calories.

10. Diets of less than 3500 kJ (800 calories) per day for women and 4200 kJ (1000 calories) per day for men should not be used unless under strict medical supervision.

11. Obese persons should be encouraged to take up gradual and extended exercise on a regular basis rather than vigorous and intermittent exercise, to supplement a dietary regime.

12. Dietary prescription for persons with known medical complications should always be carried out by a qualified nutritionist or dietition.

13. The concept of spot reduction should not be entertained in any way. All exercise should include an aerobic component if weight loss is an aim.

14. Weight control courses/programs should be able to demonstrate through written records the effectiveness of the course over both the short term (i.e. three months), and the long term (i.e. 1–2 years).

12 Nutrition for Active People

The typical Australian diet is high in fat, low in complex carbohydrate and dietary fibre, and high in salt. It is not suitable for those wanting peak performance in physical activity. It is also not suitable for those who want to minimise their risks of health problems.

No diet, however good, can of itself improve fitness. But a poor diet can certainly decrease the chances of fitness and health. A good diet, like physical activity, is a basic requirement for everyone.

Fitness oriented people need a diet which is geared much more to health than the typical Australian diet. This does not mean they need to live on grated carrots and sunflower seeds or some strange concoctions of foods. But it does mean they need to make some sensible food choices from the wide range of foods available and so produce a healthier mix of nutrients.

There are important dietary changes fitness oriented people can make. By manipulating the diet to increase complex carbohydrate, glycogen stores in muscles can be increased to extend muscular endurance. It is also helpful to reduce fats in the diet. This keeps blood fat levels low and controls the amount of body fat. It also makes sense to decrease the salt and sugar content of the diet and increase dietary fibre. Some of these changes will help athletic performance. All will assist long-term health.

Sports people are a ready target for nutrition quackery. In striving for an edge, many sportspeople take up nutrition-related practices which are useless and sometimes even counter-productive. There's nothing really new in this. The history of sport and physical fitness is riddled with stories of the superior value of particular diets and nutritional supplements. Many of the supplements said to be wonder foods for building muscle or extra energy are worthless; some will actively work against goals of achieving peak performance.

Dietary Guidelines for Australians

Australia has one of the best and most varied food supplies of any country in the world. In spite of such abundance, many people fail to make a healthy selection. Foods which are rich in complex carbohydrate and dietary fibre are often ignored and most people also fail to drink enough water. Such an eating pattern makes it difficult to achieve peak physical performance.

Some people doubt the value of the modern food supply and believe they must rely on pills for nutrients. In fact, Australia has a wonderful selection of healthy foods available and it is perfectly possible to choose an excellent diet. However, there are also many foods which are high in fat, sugar and salt and many with little or no nutritional value. The value of the diet depends on the foods you choose. The idea that the major dietary problem is a lack of vitamins is wrong. Vitamin deficiencies are rare and any diet which is so poor that it lacks vitamins will not be fixed by taking extra vitamins.

Excess weight is common in Australia. It is due to eating and drinking more kilojoules than are needed for metabolism and physical activity (and growth in children). The main culprits for most overweight people are too much fat, sugar and alcohol. Fats and sugar occur in many of our foods and slip down so effortlessly that few people realise the large amounts they are consuming. Foods such as bread, cereals, grains and potatoes are rarely responsible for excess weight. Yet it is these important sources of complex carbohydrate which many people restrict—thus making exercise difficult.

Whether you are lean or overweight, a high fat diet increases the risk of coronary heart disease, high blood pressure, diabetes, gallstones, gout, and breast and bowel cancer. Too much salt increases the chances of high blood pressure while a lack of dietary fibre upsets the functioning of the intestine and alters the body's chemical balance which controls cholesterol and glucose.

The typical Australian diet has:

- Too much fat, particularly saturated fat
- Too little complex carbohydrate
- Too little dietary fibre
- Too much sugar
- Too much salt
- Too much alcohol
- Not enough water
- Too little iron and calcium (mainly in women)
- Too much food for our level of physical activity.

The Dietary Guidelines for Australians seek to address these major problems. The guidelines are:

- Choose a nutritious diet from a variety of foods (see Table 12.1)
- Control body weight
- Avoid eating too much fat
- Avoid eating too much sugar
- Eat more breads and cereals, preferably wholegrain, and more vegetables and fruits
- Limit alcohol consumption
- Use less salt
- Promote breast feeding.

Let's take a look at some of the problem areas.

Table 12.1: The Five Food Groups

Food group	Main nutrients	Minimum daily amounts
Vegetables, fruits	Vitamin C Vitamin A (as carotene) Fibre Small amounts of many minerals and vitamins	At least 4 servings (1 piece of fruit or ½ cup vegetables = 1 serve) Choose a variety, including vitamin C-rich sources such as citrus fruits, tomato, capsicum, kiwifruit, rockmelon, strawberries and a dark green or yellow fruit or vegetable for carotene.
Breads, cereals	Thiamin Niacin Protein Some iron Fibre in wholegrain varieties	4 servings or more, depending on energy needs (1 slice bread or small bowl breakfast cereal or ½ cup pasta = 1 serve)
Meat, fish, poultry, eggs, dried beans & peas, nuts	Protein Iron Niacin Thiamin Riboflavin	1 serving (1 serve = 75–100 g meat or ¾ cup cooked beans)
Milk, cheese, yoghurt (milk can be whole, skim, evaporated or buttermilk)	Calcium Protein Riboflavin	Children & adolescents: 600 ml Adults: 300 ml Pregnancy & lactation: 600 ml (30 g cheese is equivalent to 150 ml milk)
Fats: butter or margarine	Vitamins A and D	15–30 g (1 tablespoon = 20 g)

Fat

Few people set out to eat a lot of fat but it comes with many of our favourite foods. We are now eating more fat than any previous generation of Australians. The major sources of fat in the Australian diet are as follows:

- 38% comes from oils, margarines and cooking fats (used in fast foods, fried foods, in biscuits, cakes, pastries, snack foods and many processed foods, and spread onto bread, added to vegetables and used in cooking)
- 36% comes from meat (from fatty meats, big steaks and many processed meats as well as the beef fat included in processed foods such as biscuits, pastries and fast foods)

- 15% comes from dairy products (milk, cheese, icecream and yoghurt)
- 4% comes from grain foods (hamburger buns, toasted muesli, etc.)
- 3% comes from nuts and peanut butter
- 2% comes from poultry (mainly the skin)
- 1% comes from eggs
- 1% comes from seafoods.

To cut down on fat

• Choose plenty of low fat foods such as vegetables, fruits, breads of all types, most cereals and grains and legumes.

• Avoid fried foods, pastries, biscuits and cakes most of the time.

• Use minimal quantities of butter, margarine, oil and chocolates.

• Avoid cream, mayonnaise and oily dressings.

• Avoid large serves of fatty and processed meats. Choose more seafoods, turkey or chicken (without skin) and look for lean meats such as veal, new fashioned pork, and lean cuts of beef. The leanest part of lamb is the leg.

• For fast foods, choose sandwiches, salads, toasted sandwiches, a regular hamburger, Lebanese breads filled with salad and hoummus or felafel, char-grilled barbequed chicken (leave the skin) or pizza. Try to add some fresh fruit.

• Choose some low fat dairy products such as skim, Shape or Lite White milk, non-fat yoghurt, lower fat cheeses such as cottage, ricotta, Cotto, mozzarella, Swiss or fat-reduced varieties.

Carbohydrates

Energy for fuel can be derived from proteins, fats or carbohydrates. However, carbohydrates are the muscle cell's preferred form of fuel.

Carbohydrates come in two major forms: sugars and complex carbohydrates (formerly called starches).

Sugars include:

Glucose—Mainly formed from the breakdown of all other carbohydrates. Also found in small quantities in fruits, vegetables and honey. (Glucose can also be called *dextrose*.)

Fructose—The sugar found in fruits and honey (tastes very sweet).

Galactose—A sugar resulting from the digestion of lactose in milk.

Sucrose—Regular cane sugar (made of glucose + fructose).

Lactose—Milk sugar (made of glucose + galactose).

Maltose—Malt sugar from sprouting grains (made of glucose + glucose).

The term 'sugar' is often only applied to sucrose. You may see food products with the words 'no added sugar' on the label. Check that they don't just contain some other type of sugar. Once in the body, all sugars are eventually converted to glucose. Excess quantities are stored as body fat.

Complex Carbohydrates

These are molecules made up of thousands of glucose units joined together. They occur in cereals and grains (and foods made from grains such as bread, muffins, pasta and breakfast cereals), vegetables, legumes, nuts and a few fruits (such as bananas and custard apples).

Fruits contain carbohydrate in the form of sugars. In combination with their dietary fibre, we can consider that the carbohydrate in fruits acts like the complex carbohydrates.

Most foods containing complex carbohydrates also contain dietary fibre and a range of minerals and vitamins.

Complex carbohydrate should make up 50–60% of the kilojoules in the diet.

To increase complex carbohydrate

• Eat more breads, particularly the wholemeal or wholegrain varieties.

• Eat more cereal products such as oats, wholewheat breakfast products, pasta (preferably wholemeal) and rice (preferably brown)

• Try to include grains such as barley, corn, millet, buckwheat, rye, oats, quick cook wheat and burghul.

• Eat more legumes such as lentils, soya, kidney, black-eye and other beans, chick peas and other types of dried peas.

• Include more vegetables of all types but especially potatoes.

• Use nuts as a substitute for meat sometimes.

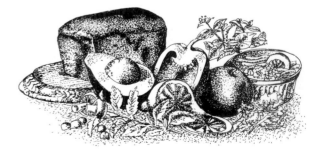

Dietary Fibre

Dietary fibre exists only in plant foods—in grains, breads and cereal products, vegetables, fruits, legumes, seeds and nuts. Animal foods have no dietary fibre. Substances are classed as 'dietary fibre' if they are not broken down by the enzymes in the small intestine.

Some types of fibre are digested by bacteria in the large intestine. It is therefore not correct to say that dietary fibre is not digested. It is simply digested in a different way from other nutrients. During the digestion of dietary fibre, bacteria multiply by the million. Their dead bodies make up more than half the weight of the faeces.

The major types of dietary fibre include:

Pectin—The type of dietary fibre found in apples, citrus peel (and marmalade), jams and fruits.

Cellulose—The 'stringy' fibre in vegetables, also found in grains and cereal foods, fruits, nuts and seeds.

Hemi-cellulose—Actually a number of related substances found in cereals and cereal products (including white bread), vegetables, fruits, nuts and seeds.

Lignin—A 'woody' type of fibre found in cereal husks, root vegetables and pears.

Polysaccharides—Carbohydrate-related substances which occur in foods such as legumes and grains.

Gums—Found in oats and legumes (dried peas and beans).

Saponins—Found in alfalfa, asparagus, chick peas, eggplant, kidney beans, mung beans, oats, peas, peanuts, soya beans, spinach and sunflower seeds.

Mucilages and gels—Usually added as thickeners in processed foods.

Early measurements of fibre only identified 'crude fibre' which represented cellulose. For this reason, old food tables which list only the crude fibre content of foods grossly underestimate the true dietary fibre content.

The old idea of fibre being 'stringy' does not apply to most types of dietary fibre. Pectin, for example, is a fine white powder which readily absorbs water. The gums in oats also absorb water to form a viscous solution rather than being an obviously coarse fibre. Foods such as celery and lettuce, where you can easily see the strings of fibre do not contribute much to dietary fibre at all. Other vegetables, legumes and grain products have much more total fibre.

When dietary fibre is being digested by bacteria in the large intestine, chemical substances known as volatile fatty acids are produced. These provide nourishment to the cells of the bowel wall. They also control muscular movement of the bowel and may have an anti-cancer effect.

Dietary fibres which are soluble in water (pectin, gums, mucilages) are almost entirely digested by bacteria and produce more of these volatile fatty acids. Rolled oats and legumes are especially useful.

Some types of fibre (gums, mucilages, pectin, saponins) also help control levels of cholesterol and glucose in the blood. They are excellent for sportspeople.

Lignin, a particularly coarse fibre, is hardly digested at all. Cellulose and the hemi-celluloses are digested to a varying extent, depending on your individual intestine and the time food remains in it.

The digestion of various types of fibre also depends on the amount present. If you eat only a small amount of cellulose, for example, most of it is digested. With a higher intake, less is broken down by the bacteria.

The physical condition of some foods is also important. Coarse bran absorbs lots of water and will pass through the large intestine faster than finely ground bran. Coarse bran forms soft faeces; fine bran forms small hard ones.

Populations who eat plenty of dietary fibre have a very low incidence of bowel cancer, diabetes, gallstones, heart disease, diverticular disease, obesity and constipation.

Constipation is a direct result of a diet which is low in fibre (and also lacks sufficient water). Most of the other conditions, however, are likely to be due to several factors, especially a high intake of fat. Foods which are high in dietary fibre are usually low in fat whereas those which are high in fat generally have little or no dietary fibre. It is therefore difficult to say whether it is the presence of fibre or the absence of fat which provides the greater benefit. It is probably both.

To increase dietary fibre

• Follow the guidelines for increasing complex carbohydrate

• Choose wholegrain products wherever possible

• Eat more fruit

• Leave skins on fruits and vegetables where practical.

Sugar

The average Australian consumes nearly 1 kg of sugar a week. More than 75% of this is already in foods. A small amount of sugar will not cause problems for most people but the average intake is certainly not 'small'. Sugar has three major disadvantages:

1. Sugar makes fats palatable (you wouldn't eat cakes, pastries, biscuits, chocolates, icecream or desserts if the sugar didn't make the fats taste nice).

2. Sugar has absolutely no vitamins, minerals, dietary fibre, protein or other essential nutrients. It is a useless product from a nutritional point of view.

3. Sugary foods can easily replace other more nutritious foods. For example, many people will eat a sweet or a chocolate bar in place of a more nutritious meal.

Major sources of sugar include:
• Soft drinks, cordials, fruit juice drinks and other sweetened drinks
• Confectionery (lollies, chocolates, sweets)
• Biscuits, cakes, pastries
• Desserts (including icecream)
• Sweetened breakfast cereals (some are nearly half sugar)
• Jams, jellies and spreads.

To cut down on sugar

• Drink water, pure fruit juices, plain mineral or soda water in place of soft drinks (or use low kilojoule soft drinks)
• Choose fresh fruit for desserts and snacks
• Avoid large quantities of cakes, pastries and biscuits
• Gradually give up sugar in tea and coffee
• Choose fruits canned without syrup
• Choose unsweetened breakfast cereals such as porridge, weetbix or other wholewheat cereals, puffed wheat or home-made muesli
• Look for jams without added sugar (avoid those with sorbitol as this contributes as many kilojoules as sugar).

Salt

The salt content of the typical diet is high. Salt is added to processed foods as well as being used in cooking and sprinkled on food at the table. Fast foods are very high in salt (most have much more salt than home-prepared food) and even items you would not think of as being salty, such as cornflakes, have a very high salt content. A bowl of cornflakes has even more salt than a packet of potato crisps.

The taste for salt is learned and by gradually using less salt, the taste buds easily adjust. Once people give up using salt, they usually find salty foods unpleasant.

Some salt is lost in sweat, but the more often you exercise, the less salt is lost. Trained athletes lose very little salt. The more salt you eat, the more water you need to drink. Most sportspeople don't drink enough water at the best of times, and a high salt intake makes any dehydration worse. Long-term, a high salt intake and also contribute to high blood pressure.

To eat less salt

• Gradually reduce the amount of salt used in cooking until you enjoy the natural flavours of foods without salt. Then reduce salt used at the table.
• Always taste food before adding salt.
• Make greater use of fresh or dried herbs for flavouring foods rather than using salt.
• Choose fresh meats rather than processed meats such as sausages, corned beef, ham, salamis etc. (except for salt-reduced varieties).
• Steam, micro-cook or stir-fry vegetables rather than boiling; the natural flavour will predominate so that you will not need salt.
• Look for unsalted canned vegetables, crackers, butter or margarine, peanut butter and other foods. Almost all canned foods come in an unsalted version.
• Choose fresh fruit or unsalted nuts or freshly popped corn instead of salty snack items.
• Choose a low salt cereal such as porridge, oats, weetbix, puffed wheat or other packet products which do not have added salt.

Alcohol

Each standard drink contains about the same amount of alcohol. Too much alcohol will adversely affect physical fitness and can damage the liver and brain. One to two drinks a day seem harmless for most people.

To cut down on alcohol
- Drink slowly.
- Have a large glass of water or mineral water before a social occasion so that the first drink is not consumed quickly to quench the thirst.
- Have water or mineral water available at meals.
- Choose low alcohol beer.

Water

Many sportspeople fail to drink sufficient water. Relying on thirst is not enough. After a heavy sweat it can take more than 48 hours for your thirst to tell you to drink enough to replace the losses. A hot climate makes this worse. Alcoholic drinks have a net negative effect on the body's water balance and cannot be considered a substitute for water. At least 6–8 glasses of water a day are needed for sedentary people.

Sportspeople need much more. Weigh yourself before and after a typical training session; the weight loss is water. You can also tell if you are drinking enough water from the colour of your urine. Except for first thing in the morning, it should be almost colourless.

Minerals

Calcium

Calcium is vitally important throughout life. The body maintains the correct level of calcium in the blood for muscle and nerve function by withdrawing or depositing calcium in the bones. A small deficit in calcium intake over the years leads to bones becoming porous causing osteoporosis.

Changes in female hormones which accompany menopause increase the loss of calcium from bones. The greater the calcium content of the bones before menopause, the lower the problem created by hormonal changes. It is therefore important for women to have plenty of calcium for many years before menopause so that the bones can withstand the stress created by ageing.

The recommended daily intake of calcium is 800 mg/day for adults. The best sources of calcium are dairy products (milk—either whole, low fat or skim, yoghurt and cheese). Fish with edible bones (sardines, tuna and salmon), almonds, soya bean milk (fortified with extra calcium) and green vegetables (not spinach) also contain calcium. Sesame seeds are not a very good source as the oxalic acid they contain forms a chemical complex with calcium making it unavailable to the body.

The amount of calcium retained in bones is decreased by a lack of female hormones (which occurs in women whose body fat level is so low that they do not menstruate), lack of exercise and a diet which is high in protein or salt.

Iron

Iron is part of haemoglobin which carries oxygen to all body tissues and takes carbon dioxide back to the lungs. In muscles, iron is an important part of myoglobin. It is also essential in the chain of chemical reactions which produce energy in the body.

A lack of iron is common in women because of blood loss every month in menstruation. Early

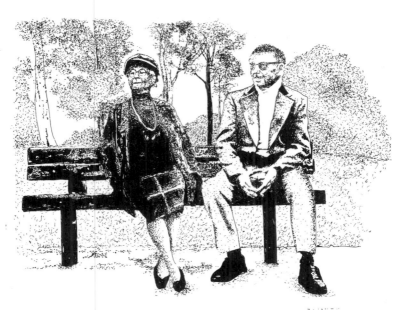

symptoms of iron deficiency include fatigue and irritability. Slimmers are at risk since most popular diets are low in iron. Iron levels can be determined by a blood test.

Men need 5–7 mg of iron a day; women need 12–16 mg—more than twice as much. During pregnancy, requirements are 22–36 mg a day.

Iron is found in oysters, red meats (especially liver and kidneys), poultry, fish, legumes, green leafy vegetables, cereals and wholemeal bread, dried fruits and eggs.

The iron in meat, seafoods and poultry is absorbed best. The iron in wholemeal bread, cereals, vegetables and eggs is absorbed to a lesser extent. Eating even a small amount of meat, fish or poultry will enhance the amount of iron absorbed from vegetables. Vitamin C, found in fruits and vegetables, also increases the absorption of iron, so it makes sense for women to eat a fruit or vegetable at each meal.

Vegetarians can obtain sufficient iron if they eat a variety of legumes, grains, seeds, nuts and vegetables. Those who simply omit most, or all, meat often become iron-deficient.

Iron supplements

It is always best to obtain nutrients from food. However, once you lack iron, supplements are a good way to correct the deficiency.

Supplements which also contain vitamin C will help the iron to be absorbed. Iron supplements should be taken with meals so that the vitamin C from the fruits and vegetables can assist absorption of the iron from the supplement.

Protein and Amino Acids

Most Australians eat plenty of protein. The average sportsperson should aim for 1 gram of protein per kilogram of body weight per day. During weight training, increase this to 1.6 g/kg. Very high levels are not desirable: excess protein is simply turned into body fat.

Proteins are made up of amino acids. Supplements of amino acids are sold to athletes in the hope that they will have an anabolic effect on muscles. To date, there is no scientifically valid research which shows that amino acids have the claimed effect. Most of the 'results' rely on anecdotal reports, usually from those who are selling the products. A small Australian study recently looked at the effect of some amino acids on the production of growth hormone (which is thought to stimulate muscle growth). They had no effect. Further scientific studies are required.

Weight Control

It is important that athletes do not carry too much body fat. Body weight itself includes bone, muscle, water and fat. Only an excessive level of body fat is undesirable.

Most slimming diets 'work' by removing water and glycogen from muscles. Many also cause a loss of muscle tissue itself. This makes it difficult to exercise and also leads to future weight gain since it is muscle tissue which burns up kilojoules. When the muscle content of the body is reduced, you may weigh less but you cannot burn up as many kilojoules (muscle burns up lots of kilojoules; fat burns hardly any). Those who try one diet after another find that they need so little food that even a normal food intake increases their body fat.

The misconception that carbohydrates are fattening occurs because low carbohydrate diets are so often recommended by popular (but usually unqualified) diet book authors. It is the sudden drop in the carbohydrate content of the diet which causes the loss of glycogen and water from the muscles. This appears as a fast loss of weight and makes slimmers believe they are successfully attacking their body fat. However, very little fat loss occurs with these diets; most of the apparent (and temporary) drop in weight comes from a loss of water.

To lose body fat
- Cut back on all types of fat.
- Avoid alcohol.
- Use little sugar.
- Include enough complex carbohydrate foods to provide glycogen so that you can exercise. Exercise will help remove body fat without losing muscle tissue.

Vitamin Supplements

Most athletes take vitamins. Few need them. If the diet is so poor that vitamins are needed, it will certainly not be providing the right balance of complex carbohydrates and other nutrients. In such cases, taking a supplement will not cure the problem. The way to correct a poor diet is to change the diet!

There is a tendency to believe that 'if a little is good, more must be better'. Some vitamin manufacturers have grown wealthy on that sort of argument.

A deficiency of vitamins (especially the B vitamins) will interfere with performance. That does not mean that extra quantities will enhance performance. It's a bit like the petrol in your car: without it, the car won't go, but if you fill the tank so that it overflows, the car does not go any better than when the tank has just enough petrol. And just as an overflowing petrol tank can damage the paintwork and be a safety hazard, so can megadoses of vitamins. Enough is enough.

The way to get enough vitamins is to eat plenty of fruits and vegetables, wholemeal bread and other cereal and grain products and to add fish, chicken or lean meat (or a vegetarian alternative).

Megadoses of some of the B complex vitamins can be detrimental to endurance athletes because they deplete glycogen stores faster.

Phony Vitamins

Vitamins B_{15}, B_{17}, B-T and P are not true vitamins. They may sell well and make money for their distributors but they have not been shown to have real benefits for athletes, apart from the belief that they will improve performance.

Other 'miracle' foods such as bee pollen, royal jelly, green magma, zell oxygen, protein powders, herbal supplements, lecithin and orotic acid also have no benefit except for those who believe in their 'magic'.

The Pre-Exercise Meal

Most people need to eat about three hours before exercise so they will neither feel hungry nor have a stomach full of food. Choose foods with carbohydrate but little fat such as bread, cereals, fruit, pasta, rice or potatoes. A large fatty meal takes 5–6 hours to be digested and is quite unsuitable.

Avoid sugar or glucose in the hour or so before exercise as it can cause a peak in blood sugar, followed by a surge of insulin and a temporary drop in blood sugar level. Weak sugar solutions (about 2.5 per cent) are suitable during endurance events. Once exercise has begun, the exercise itself controls the release of insulin.

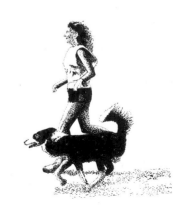

Balancing the Diet

The distribution of energy in the typical Australian diet compared with the ideal diet for physically active people is displayed in Figure 12.1.

	% Cals	
	Current diet	Ideal diet
Protein	14	10–15
Fat	40	20–30
Complex carbohydrate	15	40–55
Sugars	26	15
Alcohol	5	1

Fig. 12.1: Current Australian diet compared with dietary goals

Energy in the diet comes from proteins, fats and carbohydrates (complex and simple). Alcoholic drinks also provide energy from both the alcohol and the sugar they contain.

In order to make an approximate calculation of the percentage of energy coming from each of the nutrients, start by adding up the amount of protein, fat and carbohydrate eaten, using the figures in the tables below. Since every gram of carbohydrate or protein supplies 4 calories, and every gram of fat 9 calories, the percentage of energy coming from each nutrient can be calculated by multiplying:

• The number of grams of protein or carbohydrate by 4.
• The number of grams of fat by 9.

Add total calories and work out the percentage coming from each nutrient. For example, if estimates include 135 grams of protein, 140 grams of fat and 300 grams of carbohydrate, the calculations will be:

Protein	135 g × 4 =	540
Fat	140 g × 9 =	1260
Carbohydrate	300 g × 4 =	1200
Total calories		3000

% Protein	540/3000 × 100 = 18%
% Fat	1260/3000 × 100 = 42%
% Carbohydrate	1200/3000 × 100 = 40%

Table 12.2: Protein, fat and carbohydrate in selected foods

For further information, consult *Tables of Composition of Australian Foods,* or *Food Facts,* by Mark Wahlqvist. NB: Asterisk after carbohydrate signifies it is a sugar. Sugars and complex carbohydrates contribute an equal number of calories.

Alcohol provides 7 calories per gram. A middy of beer has 8 grams of simple carbohydrate and some 11 grams of alcohol. A glass of wine has 0.5 grams of simple carbohydrate and about 12 g alcohol.

Food	Protein	Fat	Carbohydrate
Bread/regular slice	2.0	0.5	15.0
thick slice	3.0	0.8	22.0
roll	5.0	1.0	32.0
Butter 1 tbs		15.5	
Margarine 1 tbs		15.5	
Jam 2 ts			10.0*
Sugar 1 ts			4.0*
Breakfast cereal/ average serve	2.0		23.0(*7.0)
2 Weetbix	4.0		24.0
Muesli 60 g	7.0	5.5	34.0(*13.0)
Toasted muesli 60 g	5.5	10.5	35.0(*15.0)
Milk 200 ml	7.0	8.0	10.0*
Skim milk 200 ml	7.0		10.0*
Flavoured milk 300 ml	9.0	9.0	27.0*
Cheese 30 g	8.0	10.0	
Cottage cheese 100 g	18.0	0.5	2.0
Yoghurt 200 g	9.0	7.0	12.0*
non-fat 200 g	12.0		14.0*
flavoured 200 g	12.0	7.0	34.0*
Icecream 100 ml	2.0	5.0	11.0*
Fruit/average piece	1.0		18.0*
Beans/e.g. lima	8.0	0.5	23.0*
Fruit juice 250 ml	0.5		30.0*
Vegetables salad type	0.5		2.0
cooked (average serve)	1.5		3.0
Peas ½ cup	5.0		12.0
Potato/medium	2.0		18.0
Chips/regular serve	3.0	13.0	20.0
Corn 1 cup	4.5	1.0	26.0
Pasta 1 cup	6.0		50.0
Rice 1 cup	5.0		50.0
Egg 1	6.0	6.0	
Bacon 2 strips	8.0	27.0	
Steak T-bone	50.0	46.0	
Lamb chops 2	29.0	40.0	
Sausages 2 thick	22.0	35.0	20.0
Chicken ¼ barbecued	24.0	15.0	
Fried, 2 pieces	30.0	29.0	
Hamburger	31.0	31.0	44.0(*10.0)
Small steak 100 g (no fat)	32.0	7.0	
Chicken breast 100 g	25.0	2.0	
Pizza/regular	49.0	32.0	89.0
Meat pie	13.0	24.0	31.0
Fish/grilled fillet (150 g)	27.0	4.0	
battered	21.0	23.0	20.0
Nuts 30 g	5.0	19.0	4.0
Peanut butter, 1 tbs	6.0	10.0	3.0
Oil 1 tbs		19.0	
Cakes/e.g. date loaf	4.5	7.0	35.0(*26.0)
fruitcake	3.5	9.0	35.0(*28.0)
doughnut	3.0	10.0	18.0(* 8.0)
Chocolate biscuit	1.0	5.5	14.0(*12.0)
Ryvita biscuit	1.0		8.0
Rolled oats, raw 30 g	4.0	2.0	22.0
Lentils, 1 cup cooked	12.0		24.0

13 Motivation and Maintaining Interest in Exercise

Behaviour scientists have been slow to enter the exercise field. Hence, although we know a lot about the physiology of fitness, we know very little about why people do (or don't) exercise. Yet reports show consistently that up to two-thirds of those who start an exercise program give it up within three months.

On the other hand there are those who do exercise regularly without the obvious sporting incentives of competition and success. These people often find it more difficult to miss a day's exercise than to force themselves out of bed on a cold winter morning.

The question that has to be asked is 'why'?

Why Do People Exercise?

Usually the question is asked the other way around. We're continually looking for reasons why people don't exercise, instead of looking at why millions do, daily, with no obvious reward.

What makes non-competition runners, for example, go to great lengths to avoid missing a day pounding the streets? What makes tennis players with little or no basic talent risk the aches and pains of the day-after to beat a ball around a court? What makes surfers put up with freezing winter conditions to risk getting driven into the sand by an oversized wave?

The answer of course is enjoyment, although to many this may seem a little hard to believe. There's likely to be little enjoyment for somebody beginning to exercise a previously sedentary body. This will only come as the level of fitness improves to the point that physical activity becomes, as it should be, a natural human activity.

As well as this, there are individual differences in motivation. For some, the initial motivation to exercise may be to look better, feel healthier, ward off sickness or delay the onset of ageing. Others are more caught up in the tide of social fashion; they start exercising because others are doing it; even though they may *continue* to exercise at a later point because it becomes enjoyable.

All this suggests that the motivation to exercise is dynamic as well as individualistic. What serves to motivate some beginning exercisers will not necessarily work for others, and what motivates the beginner may not be necessary for the more advanced.

Indeed, stages of fitness have been identified at which the sources of motivation may vary significantly. The fitness leader needs to be aware of these from the early stages of the reluctant exerciser to the more advanced stage of the exercise addict.

Stages of Fitness

There now seems to be general agreement among behavioural scientists that any previously inactive person who begins an exercise program will go through a series of motivational stages.

The first of these is a 'mild discomfort' stage where

any increased effort is, as it implies, mildly discomforting. This can last for anything from 2 to 10 weeks, and requires a good deal of time and effort on the part of a motivator to see it through.

The second, or 'physical' stage is where the exercise

stops hurting and even begins to feel good—at least after each session. But there's still little intrinsic or internal reward from the exercise itself.

Some people only get this far. And that's enough. The rewards of feeling and looking better are quite often more than enough to keep someone coming back for those same feelings.

Others can reach a third or psychological stage where the exercise is rewarding—even while it's being carried out. It becomes almost a form of meditation as the mind relaxes and transcends mundane daily events and the body moves into a 'flow' or easy movement pattern. At this stage the exerciser can become hooked and it's no longer necessary for outside or extrinsic motivation to keep him or her going.

The stages of fitness, their characteristics and the type of motivation required to ensure adherence at each stage are shown in Figure 13.1.

The aim of any exercise program should be to get the individual from stage 1 or the level of extrinsic motivation to stage 3 or the level of intrinsic motivation.

Extrinsic and Intrinsic Motivation

The terms extrinsic and intrinsic are used to define the level of internality required in a reward system. Extrinsic reward is that which is outside or not inherent in the individual. It includes such incentives as working to a points system, for financial gain, for social acclaim.

Intrinsic reward on the other hand comes from within or is inherent in the individual. This includes feelings of well-being, achievement, satisfaction or mental enhancement.

Intrinsic reward (and motivation) generally comes from the individual performing the task. There is little need for an outside person or motivator. Extrinsic reward is usually offered by an individual for him or herself, or by another person or external motivator.

Stage	Characteristics	Motivation
1. Discomfort	anaerobic; mild discomfort, lack of wind, desire to stop	extrinsic, cosmetic, health, social, financial
2. Physical	aerobic/anaerobic; feeling of physical wellbeing, wind easy but no feeling of flow	ex/intrinsic—physical gains, health benefits, social status, fit feeling
3. Psychological	aerobic; feeling of flow, enjoyment during the effort, mental relaxation, exhilaration, increase in creativity	intrinsic—mental wellbeing, relaxation, enjoyment, 'escape'

Fig. 13.1: Stages of Fitness

Motivating Through the Stages

Stages 1 and 2 described above call for an extrinsic reward system and hence are times at which an instructor can be most helpful. In stage 3, the instructor can play a lesser role as the exercise takes on its own reward. This is the stage at which runners talk of a 'runner's high', and others refer to an 'addiction to exercise'.

Not everyone will reach this third level. But for those with the capability, there are certain extrinsic techniques which can be used to help the progression through stages 1 and 2.

Stage 1: Discomfort

Any sedentary person starting an exercise program will feel minor discomfort after an exercise session. This can be minimised by the correct training procedures and exercise principles, but the feeling of sore muscles after exercise is unlikely to drive the exerciser back for more.

The length of time taken to pass through this stage will depend on a number of factors, including the basal level of fitness of the individual. It may take from 2 weeks to 6 months. However, the client should be made aware that things will improve. Motivation techniques to help through this stage include:

Using the 'Mate' System: Individuals can be paired with a person of similar interests and fitness to help decrease the chances of exercise avoidance.

Recording Progress: Records of improvements towards short-term and long-term goals should be kept in a prominent position in easily readable form. These may include charts of heart rate, body measurements, fitness tests, or of calorific usage.

Rewarding Effort: Individual exercise efforts can be rewarded by both the instructor and the individual exerciser. Cooper's Aerobic Points system (see *Aerobics* and *The New Aerobics*) provides a method of record and reward which serves to reinforce the exerciser for his/her efforts. Other rewards in the gym include club membership, certificates, clothing and other incentives for best improvements over set time periods.

Encouraging: Perhaps the most successful, but often overlooked, form of reinforcement is encouragement and praise from a respected source. The instructor is invariably in a position to offer such encouragement.

Creating Awareness: Individuals need to be made aware of the stages of fitness and the progression they are likely to make through a planned exercise program. If it's thought that exercise will offer a 'high' from day 1, clients will quickly become disillusioned.

Emphasising Short-Term Goals: Although long-term goals are often the purpose of an exercise program, short-term goals are likely to be more immediately rewarding. Instead of aiming to lose 10 kg of body weight overall, a more realistic short-term goal would be to lose 0.5 kg per week.

Using Variety: Variety can be a potent way of maintaining interest, particularly with the beginning exerciser. A mixed program of exercise can serve to allow the beginner the opportunity to choose a preferred exercise mode for long-term use, reduce boredom and assist in the prevention of stress injuries from over-use of one particular muscular or skeletal group.

Planning Ahead: There are many different types of aerobic exercise and individuals are suited to each of these depending on their body build, attitudes, interests and abilities. Often, the most appropriate exercise is only chosen after experience with that exercise. In the long term, it is only exercise that is enjoyable for the individual which will have prospects of becoming a lifestyle habit.

Encouraging the Use of Fantasy and Imagination: One of the main benefits of exercise often stressed by psychologists is its value as a form of time out from other aspects of life. To this extent, many find exercise a useful form of mental relaxation where fantasy, imagination and creativity come to the fore. Rehearsal, where the planned exercise effort is continuously imagined before it is carried out, is another technique of increasing motivation.

Establishing a Contract: This can be drawn up with the client and based on a commitment to carry out exercise at a certain level over a set period of time. The document should be in writing, and referred to whenever necessary!

Stage 2: Physical Reward

Stage 2 is physical reward from exercise. Many people can reach this level after only a short period of regular exercise and many don't progress beyond it. Once the feelings of well-being that come from exercise have been reached, the main aim of a motivator is to maintain adherence to a program. The motivational aims thus move from encouraging initiation to improving maintenance.

According to Professor John Martin, an expert in the behavioural management of exercise from the University of Mississippi Medical Centre, there are a number of factors which predict drop-outs or poor adherers to an exercise program. These are summarised under 4 headings:

Subject Factors: Adherence is lower amongst those people who:
- Are smokers
- Have low self motivation
- Are inactive in their leisure time
- Are overweight
- Are blue collar workers
- Have a poor credit rating.

Program Factors: Poorer results are reported for programs with:
- An inconvenient location
- High intensity exercise
- A lack of feedback
- A preoccupation with the body
- Exercise alone
- Calisthenics as their main base
- Inflexible goals.

Consequent Factors: There is a decrease in adherence resulting from:
- Injury

- An unsupportive partner/instructor
- A low level of enjoyment.

Other Factors: Declines in maintenance also occur as a result of:

- The weather (cold/rain etc.)
- Competing activities
- A job change or move
- Vacations or travel.

One way of encouraging greater adherence, according to Martin, is to reduce the potency of these factors. If clients are taught self-management techniques such as self-monitoring, goal-setting, behavioural contracts, self-instruction and rehearsal, greater adherence can also be expected.

Stage 3: The Psychological Factor

Stage 3 is a level of intrinsic reward where the exercise is motivated by the feelings of mental well-being associated with exercise. These can include states of altered consciousness, relaxation, loss of ego awareness, distortion of time perception and heightened feelings. For a further description of this stage see Egger (1981).

At this level, little extrinsic motivation is needed to encourage the individual to exercise. Indeed the exercise itself can become somewhat addictive.

Exercise as Addiction

The addictive nature of exercise was demonstrated by Dr Frederick Baekland from the University of California in 1970. Baekland offered a group of

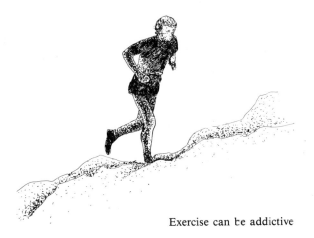

Exercise can be addictive

runners substantial financial rewards to refrain from running for two months in order to test the effects of exercise deprivation among habitually active people.

No regular runners would volunteer, so Baekland was forced to use runners who exercised only every other day. Still, these runners showed classic symptoms of withdrawal—irritability, tension, guilt, anxiety, frustration—during their time of inactivity.

Exercise and 'Flow'

In another line of research, University of Chicago psychologist Mihalyi Csikzentmihalyi has studied intensively behaviours that are autotelic or self-rewarding. These include exercise, sports, games and other intensively involving pastimes. Csikzentmihalyi concludes that all of these activities can involve mental states which can be satisfying and transcending. The doer of the activity achieves a mental state referred to as 'flow', because this best describes the feelings of the doer.

According to Csikzentmihalyi, flow is dependent on two main parameters—one related to task difficulty, the other to the competence of the performer. This is summarised in Figure 13.2.

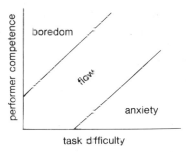

Fig. 13.2: 'Flow' and Performance (from Csikzentmihalyi, 1975)

In a situation where the difficulty of the task exceeds the competence of the person carrying out that task, a situation of anxiety arises. For example, a moderately competent mountain climber faced with a grade A slope is unlikely to settle comfortably into a flow pattern, but is more likely to be anxious in that situation.

On the other hand, a highly competent performer faced with an easy task is likely to become bored. A grade A climber on a grade C slope has less stimulation than necessary to require full concentration and is therefore mentally unoccupied as well as physically unconcerned.

The same is true of an individual in an exercise program. If the exercise is too easy for that person's level of condition it will be boring; if it's too hard it will be stressful. Either way, it will serve to demotivate the individual.

Exercise as a Drug

The flow pattern of physical activity is the level at which the exerciser can develop an attachment to exercise that has similarities with drug addiction. The difference for most people is, as William Glasser points out in his book *Positive Addictions*, that exercise is generally a positive addiction. It is controlled by the individual and enhances that person's life. However, like excessive drug use, it can become a 'negative addiction', such that it controls an individual's life and can detract from it.

The runner who continues to run through the pain of a chronic stress injury is an example of a negative addict. This is exemplified by the case of a 35-year-old university professor cited by Dr Bill Morgan in *Runner* magazine. He began running 'because everybody else was doing it', but soon began to get positive rewards despite leg injuries.

'Even though I learned to work through the pains during my runs,' he claimed, 'the pain following my runs became more and more excruciating. I had to walk downstairs backwards in the morning. I knew something was wrong, but I could just not give it up—it felt too good, it meant too much—I had to have it.'

Over-Motivation

The fitness leader needs to be aware of the symptoms of negative addiction ('over-motivation'). Over-training can be seriously debilitating and can show up in the form of chronic injuries (stress fractures, tendinitis, persistent pain); loss of interest in work, family, other hobbies etc; a deterioration in general fitness levels and appearance, even though training is occurring at a high level; and a single-minded dedication to training quantity in contrast to quality.

In an article published in the *New England Journal of Medicine* in 1983, a group of University of Arizona psychiatrists compared the 'obligatory' exerciser, particularly runners, with the compulsion of Anorexia Nervosa sufferers. The two types of people, they claim, have similar negative addictions.

According to the Arizona group, the typical obligatory runner is an exercise-conscious man in the third to fifth decade of his life. The typical anorexic is a diet-conscious women in late adolescence or early 20s. Both report a subjective 'high' from their experiences and carry out their activities with minimal pain or hunger.

While this view is far from proven, the notion of an obligatory or negatively addicted exerciser brings home the point that extremes of anything can be dangerous. Where the negative effects of any exercise begin to outweigh the positive, the rescheduling of priorities may be necessary. In the first place, a serious attempt should be made to limit the type and amount of exercise being carried out. Where the amount can't be restricted, a change of type of exercise may help to reduce the addiction.

14 Stress Management and Relaxation

Many people consider taking up an exercise program not just because of declining physical fitness, but also because they are suffering from stress. They feel that a fitness leader can help to alleviate or at least reduce the problem.

Yet not only are fitness leaders ill-equipped to deal with stress, so too are many psychologists and psychiatrists. This is understandable, because the subject of stress is complicated and confusing. Unlike exercise, it's also an area where individual responses do not invariably predict a standard outcome.

Policemen, politicians and test pilots, for example, thrive on a high level of stress. Others suffer physical and psychological ailments from pressures which, to an outsider, at least, don't appear to be stressful at all.

How much do we know about stress? More particularly, what are the known ways of coping with it? In this chapter we look at some of the answers.

What is Stress?

Stress is the 'non-specific' response of a body which finds itself under 'attack'. It is an unavoidable aspect of life which most people handle adequately most of the time.

According to Professor Hans Selye, the Canadian endocrinologist, acknowledged as one of the world's leading experts on the subject, *stress itself is not a problem*. The stress reaction is perfectly normal. It prepares the body to cope with the situation confronting it by increasing heart rate and adrenalin and preparing the muscles for action; in other words for 'fight' or 'flight'.

'Flight' is the action of escaping from that which is provoking the stress; 'fight' means tackling it head on. These days, usually neither response is entirely appropriate. Running away is not always possible, and fighting not always advisable. But the same physical reactions occur nonetheless, leaving the body to 'stew in its own juices' as it were.

'Stress', says Selye, 'depends not on what happens to an individual, but upon the way he reacts'.

Physical Symptoms

At the extremes, stress can present in the form of disease, such as in allergies, asthma, chronic fatigue, heart disease, insomnia, ulcers, bowel problems, depression, palpitations, impotence or mental illness. More commonly it can show up in muscle tightness and soreness, and general anxiety. In response to stress the large 'preparatory' muscles of the body (trapezius, gluteals, abdominals, lower back) become tense and ready for 'fight' or 'flight'. If these are not then relaxed through appropriate action of some kind, they can remain tense, causing strain and pain. It's this reaction which is found most commonly in individuals who look to fitness work for relief.

Everyone *seeks* some level of stress. If stress is absent altogether, boredom sets in, and neurosis, dissatisfaction and psychological disturbances can occur. If the stress level is too high, physical disease is likely to materialise in addition to psychological disturbance.

Yet even in the same person, it seems, reaction to stress can vary markedly over time. A Swedish group of researchers has shown for example that hormone levels indicative of stress can build up gradually in workers who put in a lot of overtime.

This shows the importance of weekends and holidays in breaking the stress cycle. It also points to two key aspects that are often over-looked in preventing and dealing with the problem—*control* and *escape*.

Control: The Key

The level of stress with which an individual seems able to cope appears to be related to that person's ability to feel in control of a situation. The politician or test pilot for example can cope with high levels of stress so long as they are in control. As soon as the former loses power, or the latter's plane goes into an uncontrollable nosedive, stress can follow. Life that may have been a 'breeze' up to that point, suddenly becomes disturbingly arousing.

Similar things happen to everyone daily. The individual caught in a traffic jam and running late for an important meeting can be highly stressed if he/she can't get to a phone. If a phone is accessible, control is restored and the situation is no longer stressful.

Psychologist Martin Seligman has shown in his book *Helplessness* that if a loss of control over one's life develops, a situation of 'learned helplessness' can arise. This can lead to a spiral of stress resulting in a wide variety of symptoms. Seligman has shown in animals that even death can result.

Researchers also point out that much drug abuse comes from what they call a psychological CHASM, which is an acronym for:

- Control loss
- Helplessness
- Alienation
- Specific circumstances
- Meaninglessness

Restoring control is often difficult, particularly if external pressures are severe. Some helpful techniques, however, include:

- Building up resistance by regular sleep, exercise and good nutrition
- Withdrawing physically from a stressful situation for a while
- Taking regular holidays
- Recognising optimal stress levels and not exceeding them
- Avoiding situations involving ambiguity and uncertainty
- More efficient time planning
- Learning a technique of mental 'escape' for occasions when this can't be done physically.

Escape: The Second Key

When stress is a recurring problem, an appropriate reaction is 'escape'. This doesn't simply mean running away, as in the 'flight' reaction of the past, but may refer to a mental response. Some physical and mental escapes are listed in Table 14.1.

Some individuals are best suited to the mental approach, some to the physical. To determine which is more appropriate, Harvard University psychologist Dr Gary Schwartz has developed a 'Stress Type Test' (see Table 14.2).

Table 14.1: Mental and Physical Escapes from Stress

Physical	Mental
Exercise	Meditation
Sport	Muscle relaxation
Warm baths	Prayer
Holidays	Concentration
Hobbies	Art
Games	Mind games
Yoga	Music

Table 14.1 cont'd

Tai-Chi	Philosophy
Martial arts	Creativity
Dancing	Reading
Talking	Theatre
Sunbathing	Trance

Table 14.2: Stress Type Test

Instructions: Circle a number from one to five for each symptom, one meaning 'not at all' and five, 'very much so'.

	Not at all				Very much so
a. I find it difficult to concentrate because of uncontrollable thoughts	1	2	3	4	5
b. I worry too much over something that doesn't matter	1	2	3	4	5
c. My heart beats faster	1	2	3	4	5
d. I imagine terrifying scenes	1	2	3	4	5

Table 14.2 cont'd

e. I get diarrhoea	1	2	3	4	5
f. I can't keep anxiety-provoking thoughts out of my mind	1	2	3	4	5
g. I feel jittery in my body	1	2	3	4	5
h. I pace nervously	1	2	3	4	5
i. I feel like I'm losing out on things because I can't make my mind up soon enough	1	2	3	4	5
j. I become immobilised	1	2	3	4	5

Scoring:
Add up the score on each of the 2 scales below.
Mental = A+B+D+F+I =
Physical = C+E+G+H+J =

Those who rank most highly on mental response should be more suited to techniques outlined below in sections 1 and 2. Those who score highest on physical response should be more suited to the physical techniques listed in 3. Where available, resources for learning the techniques are specified.

Stress Management Techniques

1. Mental Relaxation

This can include the following:

Concentration: Many relaxation techniques involve concentration. The best-known are yoga and meditation. Others include sports such as the martial arts. The main forms of concentration are on breathing, vision, resolve, mantras and muscular tension.

Concentrated Breathing: Again, many different techniques are used, including simply listening to the breath, counting whilst breathing, alternate nostril breathing and diaphragmatic breathing. Most of these are derived from yoga practices and can be found in popular instruction manuals on eastern relaxation techniques.

Visual Concentration: Breathing can be combined with techniques of visual concentration such as focusing on an object without permitting oneself to be distracted unduly. The object may be a flower, or a scene. The visual image is studied in depth by becoming absorbed in it.

Resolve Concentration. This means selecting a positive statement and mentally repeating it; for example, a statement signalling intent to escape from a stressful situation, such as 'I will think positively about work and not be bothered by minor stressful situations'. This technique can also involve processes such as 'thought stopping', where the individual is taught to practice *not to think* obsessively about a bothersome thought or unimportant detail. These approaches can be found in any behaviour modification text.

Mantra Concentration: A mantra is a word repeated mentally in order to block out thoughts which may be distracting. Mantras are generally chosen from meaningless syllables so that concentration is not diverted.

Meditation is the main form of mantra concentration. While many religions involve varieties of meditation (which can include prayer), meditation principles can be learned outside a religious context. Many health departments and private courses teach meditation over short terms at low cost.

2. Physical/Mental Relaxation

Some techniques involve aspects both of physical and mental escape, e.g.:

Progressive Muscular Relaxation: Progressive muscular relaxation (PMR) works on the principle that if the body is relaxed, the mind must be also. PMR uses conscious control of all the large muscles of the body, and while there are many versions of the technique, all involve learning to relax at will. They can also include concentration on breathing and the use of visual imagery. Typically, the individual is asked to concentrate on the small muscles of the feet, then legs, then hips, then trunk etc., until the whole body is progressively relaxed.

Most community health centres now teach PMR and in many cases audio tapes are available for purchase. Commercial PMR training should be approached with caution because of the high costs involved. They are not necessary. Reference works such as *Relief Without Drugs* by Dr Ainslie Meares are valuable sources of information.

Yoga: There are many types emphasising progressions, such as *Pranayama* (rhythmic control of the breath), *Asana* (posture), *Dhyana* (meditation) and *Dharana* (concentration).

Perhaps the most common in the West is *Hatha Yoga*, which comprises breathing techniques and physical exercises. *Raja Yoga* involves meditative practices similar to those outlined above, but with less emphasis on the physical aspects. *Raja* is generally used as a progression from *Hatha Yoga* because of the level of concentration required. *Iyengar* is a very disciplined practice, and is often recommended for the advanced student. It entails breathing techniques combined with yoga postures. In this case, breathing enhances relaxation gained by body awareness and various positions.

Academies and private schools which teach some or all of the above yoga techniques exist throughout Australia. Much literature is available on the subject.

3. Physical Relaxation

Finally, there are physical forms of relaxation such as aerobic exercise. For many, such as the Type A personality and otherwise busy people, exercise is a definite aid to relaxation. As we have seen, it also has the added advantage of aiding heart/lung conditioning, weight control, and health generally.

15 Special Problems and Exercise Instruction

Most exercise theory is based on the principle that the exerciser is 'normal'. Yet surveys show that up to 80% of the population suffer one or more forms of disability, ranging from minor respiratory ailments to paraplegia.

The more severe types of disability require individualised, specialist attention. However, many other common ailments are encountered by the fitness leader in any large population. These include the following:

Allergies to Exercise

Allergic reactions to exercise were relatively unheard of in the past. But with increasing numbers participating in fitness classes, the problem is becoming more common.

Symptoms

In a recent review of exercise-related allergies, a team of University of Minnesota allergists headed by Dr William Eisenstadt classify these under 3 headings:

- Exercise-induced anaphylaxis (allergic 'shock')
- Exercise-related forms of urticaria ('nettlerash')
- Exercise-induced asthma.

Most common symptoms of the first 2 are pruritis (itchiness), skin rashes, swelling; occurring most commonly in runners, but also in those carrying out other sustained vigorous activities. In severe cases, anaphylaxis may be life-threatening, such as with allergies to bee stings, penicillin, etc. Other symptoms can include heart-beat irregularities, stomach and nervous system upset, repeated coughing and lowered blood pressure.

Symptoms usually begin about 5 minutes after starting to exercise, but might not occur until after it is over. Also, they don't necessarily occur after every exercise session. Generally the reactions subside after 30 minutes to 4 hours, but headaches can last several days in some cases.

Causes

The causes, in most cases, aren't known. But the reaction is more common in individuals who are generally allergic, together with those with a familiy tendency to exercise-induced allergy.

Asthma is common in about 10% of the population (see below), but with proper medication can be well controlled. However, allergists point out that exercise-induced asthma can also occur in otherwise non-asthmatic individuals as a result of a reaction to certain food or drugs taken before exercise: aspirin for example can lead to severe shortness of breath and wheezing. But it's not known how common this reaction is.

Tips for the Fitness Leader

Where an obvious reaction to exercise occurs, fitness leaders should look for a 'pattern' in the preceding 12–24 hours.

Headaches after morning exercise where only coffee is taken beforehand, for example, implicate coffee (or perhaps an ingredient of coffee such as caffeine) directly as the culprit. In other cases, an allergy to a particular type of solid food (e.g. shellfish, cheese, celery, etc.) may also show up after vigorous exercise. In less common cases, *any* food eaten within 2 hours of exercise can cause a reaction.

Outdoors, allergies to grasses or pollens can become more severe with exercise. And these can even have cross-reactions with certain foods or drinks. The Minnesota team point out that chamomile tea can cross-react with certain grass allergies if drunk immediately before exercise. Beer and honey are also foods with cross-reaction potential.

In indoor exercise classes, there might be allergic reaction to dust on carpeted floors. Cross-reactions are also possibe here, but these are not clearly understood yet.

Food allergies can be systematically and safely checked by eliminating either the suspected food from the diet, or re-introducing foods one at a time after a 24-hour fast. If this is not successful, an allergist should be consulted. Medication may be necessary. In severe cases where cause can't be found and there's no reaction to medication, the only option might be to modify the type or duration of exercise program.

Anorexia

Anorexia is a condition characterised by severe underweight and an obsession by the sufferer to remain extremely thin. This is generally effected by self-starvation. With the increased social acceptance of exercise, more cases of anorexia are now being seen in gyms and fitness classes.

The disease is most common in women under 30 and seems to be caused by a psychological problem resulting from a struggle to establish a sense of control and identity. As most sufferers come from a comfortable middle-class background, parental relationships seem to play some part in the problem.

Anorexia is characterised by weight loss, ammenorhoea (cessation of periods), and other effects of starvation including reductions in metabolic rate, body temperature, pulse and blood pressure, increases in anaemia and sleep disturbances. Anorexics typically don't see themselves as abnormally thin, but take pleasure in extreme weight loss. They won't admit hunger and often develop bizarre eating habits such as avoiding foods believed to be 'fattening', not eating at all for long periods, or eating only a limited range of foods.

Diuretics and laxatives are often used to reduce body fluids and weight, and if the anorexic does occasionally give in to eating binges, this is compensated for by self-induced vomiting.

Anorexics come to fitness classes looking for exercise programs to help them stay thin. Because of their enthusiasm and denial of their condition, it's often difficult to convince them that extreme exercise may not be advisable.

Tips for the Fitness Leader

Individuals more than 20% under ideal weight should be advised to get medical approval before starting an exercise program.

In many cases, anorexics are unaware that they are dangerously underweight. This often needs to be pointed out in a firm manner, and the possible hazards explained. However, as one of the main characteristics of the disease is denial of the problem, the subject has to be approached cautiously.

Anorexia is a psychological infirmity. Correction requires extended and expert treatment which is available in most major hospitals. The role of the fitness leader should be to act as a point of first contact rather than as an immediate source of treatment or advice.

Anorexia is unlikely to be as widespread a problem as obesity in affluent societies. Nevertheless, some experts believe it may exist in up to 1% of adolescent girls, making it common enough to warrant attention by fitness leaders.

Arthritis

Although it takes many forms, arthritis is basically an inflammation around the joints. The causes are varied and not well understood, and treatments are primarily symptom-oriented. The symptoms are pain and loss of movement, followed by swelling and a change in the shape of the joint.

Rheumatoid arthritis is more common among the 20–55 age group, and women are 3 times more liable to suffer from it than men. Osteoarthritis occurs as part of the ageing process. It happens mainly in weight-bearing joints (hips, knees and spine) and can be associated with previous injury.

Arthritis and Exercise

Although exercise is likely to help the arthritic patient in increasing mobility as well as in improving general health, it should never be thought that excessive exercise will overcome the problem. Prescription should include regular stretching and strengthening exercises, with a progression to more dynamic aerobic activities once pain has begun to subside. Sometimes the exercise effect can be assisted by pain-relieving heat or cold therapy, or through stretching within the comfort of a heated pool. Stretching can progress from static to active-assisted to active as improvement occurs.

Strengthening exercises can help reduce the effects of immobilisation of a joint. They can also reverse the deteriorating co-ordination effects of agonist and antagonist muscles. Isometric exercises in the early stages are probably best, with isotonic activities being introduced as the symptoms of the disease begin to improve.

Arthritics can also benefit from aerobic exercise, but fatigue and increased stress on an affected joint should be avoided. For this reason, weight-bearing exercises such as swimming and cycling are preferable to jogging for long term improvements. Most experts agree that although jogging does not predispose to arthritis in the healthy individual, it is probable that repetitive jarring on hard pavements will accelerate damage in the arthritic joints of the lower limbs.

Asthma

Around 5% of the population are known to suffer from asthma. However, surveys with Australian school-children have shown that when faced with an asthmatic irritant, around 10% of coastal youngsters and 12.4% of country children suffer asthma. Still, asthmatics are often over-represented in sporting and fitness activities. Around 15% of the Australian Olympic swimming team which went to Moscow in 1980 were asthmatic.

This is not, however, surprising. Experts agree that improved fitness will increase the breathing capacity of the asthmatic and reduce the need for drugs. Other research has made the asthmatic's involvement in fitness programs a vital part of therapy.

What is Asthma?

Asthma is a breathing disorder caused by constriction of the air ducts in the lungs. It generally runs in families and results from an over-sensitivity of lining mucous membrane and muscles of air ducts. The air ducts react to specific irritants such as house dust, pollens, animals, nervous tension, or smog and fumes. In most cases, asthma is also brought on by vigorous exercise. It was once thought that the majority of children with asthma would grow out of it, but surveys have now shown that up to 50% can be still symptomatic at adulthood.

The exact causes of asthma aren't known. However, it's now suspected that changes in the sensitivity of the air ducts are caused by moisture losses in the airways related to ventilation and cooling. For this reason it's thought that asthmatics will react more adversely to exercise in dry conditions. Research by Australian Olympic team physician Dr Ken Fitch has verified this in showing less reaction by asthmatics to swimming than other aerobic sports such as running or cycling. The asthma sufferer will also usually react worse to exercise in cold conditions (e.g. winter mornings) or at altitude, because the air in these conditions is dry.

Jogging on the other hand may expose the asthmatic to allergens such as pollens and smog, which can trigger a reaction.

Exercise and Asthma

Modern medications have made exercise easy and advisable for asthmatics. Aerosol sprays such as *Ventolin* act as bronchial relaxants and, if used before exercise, can prevent an asthmatic attack.

With continuous and gradual exercise the asthmatic can develop greater respiratory muscle tone and so reduce the need for medication. The best types of exercise here are aerobic and those that encourage greater respiration through resistance (e.g. weight training such as bench press, pull overs etc.).

Care should be taken to ensure an adequate and gradual warm-up, particularly in cold conditions. Because winter air is coldest (and therefore usually driest) in the early morning, the asthmatic may find exercising easier on winter afternoons.

Tips for the Fitness Leader

In designing an exercise program for an asthmatic, the following should be taken into consideration:

- Avoid exercises that necessitate lying on dusty floors or carpets which could contain allergenic substances like house dust, animal hair etc.
- Advise the client to take oral medication before, and if necessary during, an exercise session. If this doesn't give relief the exercise should be discontinued.
- Include aerobic exercises and those which would encourage the use of the respiratory muscles. These may include weight training, interval training, breathing exercises etc.
- If possible encourage the client to take up swimming or water exercises, where inhaled air is warm and moist.
- Be sensitive to the fact that up to ⅓ of children in an exercise program may show some symptoms of asthma (e.g. coughing heavily after exercise). This should be acted on by reducing the exercise load and seeking medical advice.
- Encourage those with chronic wheezing or coughing after exercise to get medical attention. Medication may reverse the effects, but lack of medication can lead to chronic lung damage.
- Encourage exercise in the moister times of the day, e.g. afternoons rather than cold (dry) winter mornings.

Exercise Anaemia

In general, the scientific literature leans away from advocating vitamin and mineral supplements for athletes and heavy exercisers—provided that they eat a varied and balanced diet.

But one issue on which advise is more divided is that of iron. Are there possible deficiencies of iron in endurance athletes (particularly women and adolescents), and will iron supplements help?

The Function of Iron

Iron ('haem') is contained in a protein molecule ('globin') called *haemoglobin* which exists in red blood cells in the bloodstream. Protein and iron combine like a motorcycle and sidecar. Without the sidecar an extra passenger couldn't be transported: without iron, the globin couldn't carry oxygen to the working muscles

of the body because iron is needed to bind oxygen chemically.

A decrease in haemoglobin in the bloodstream can lead to low oxygen utilisation, resulting in constant tiredness and low energy. The condition is called 'anaemia', which simply means 'lack of blood'. The anaemic person can generally be identified by paleness around the mouth, whiteness of the blood vessels of the eyes, and a pervasive feeling of tiredness. It has been estimated that about 2–3% of Australian adults may be anaemic.

There is also an indication that heavy exercise may decrease haemoglobin levels in some people because of either:

(a) An increase in total blood volume which occurs with endurance exercise and which isn't matched by an increase in haemoglobin.

(b) Reduced haemoglobin production resulting

from low iron stores. Although the reason for the low iron observed in some athletes (e.g. runners) isn't known, it could be through:

1. Low iron in the diet
2. Low absorption of iron in the digestive tract
3. High rates of iron loss.

(c) A breakdown of the red blood cells (which carry haemoglobin) through physical trauma.

Yet although some surveys of athletes have shown haemoglobin levels around the lower level of what is regarded as the normal range (i.e. 15 g/100 ml), there's little indication that this would cause problems. *Unless they have an extremely poor diet it's unlikely that iron levels in most exercisers should cause any concern.*

Two possible exceptions to this are:

1. Heavily exercising women (particularly vegetarians who have had children).
2. Highly active adolescents who may be on poor and hence low iron diets.

The problem may be exaggerated in women because of heavy blood (and hence haemoglobin) losses in menstruation, and in adolescents because of extra iron needed during the growth spurt.

Tips for the Fitness Leader

If anaemia is suspected in an exerciser, he/she should be referred for a blood test, and medical advice if necessary. Women in the at-risk category should be advised to have a blood test at least annually.

Iron poisoning is possible (although unlikely with the doses recommended in most supplements). Hence *iron supplements without medical advice are never advisable.* In any case, studies have shown that supplements don't significantly increase haemoglobin in those with normal levels.

Individuals at risk or suspected of anaemia can be advised to eat a diet high in iron, protein, vitamin B12 and vitamin C. Good foods in these categories are leafy vegetables and organ meats like liver and kidney. Vegetarians may need a vitamin B12 supplement.

Because vitamin C helps the absorption of iron, foods high in both C and iron (leafy vegetables and citrus fruits) should be encouraged.

Diabetes

Diabetes affects about 3% of the adult population. But the incidence of the disease is rapidly rising, to the extent that estimates suggest that up to 5% of the adult population could be sufferers by the turn of the century.

There are two possible reasons for this:

First, there is an increasing proportion of aged in the population (and at least one type of diabetes is age-related). Second, there are now more diabetics being born because the disease is inherited and medical advances have meant that diabetics can now survive to reproduction age where they might not have in the past.

In terms of management, it is now accepted that regular aerobic exercise has a positive effect on the body's sensitivity to insulin (the hormone that allows glucose to be used as fuel). By maintaining a regular exercise program, the diabetic is thus thought to be able to balance the large fluctuations in blood sugars that are known to occur in diabetes.

Diabetes is a complex medical disorder which exists in two forms, both of which are caused by abnormalities of insulin. One form occurs in young people (juvenile onset diabetes) and is related to a deficiency of the pancreas in producing insulin. The other begins late in life (adult onset diabetes), and is due to an insufficiency of insulin action.

Normally, insulin helps cells to 'burn' or metabolise glucose from the blood, as oxygen helps burn wood in a fire. Because the diabetic's supply of insulin is retarded, blood glucose (sugars) remain high or fluctuate rapidly, and body cells begin to 'starve' of energy. As a result, the diabetic easily tires, feels weak, and begins to lose weight rapidly as the body's cells are starved. Other symptoms are *polydipsia* (thirst), *polyphagia* (incessant hunger) and *polyuria* (frequent urination).

In most cases of juvenile onset diabetes, regular daily insulin injections are required to balance blood sugar levels, but in some adult onset cases, dietary management is enough. This means a controlled intake of sugary foods and excess calories (if the patient is obese). In some cases where insulin is used, it's possible to misjudge and use an excess amount resulting in a *too low* blood sugar level (hypoglycaemia), which can cause light-headedness, lack of judgment, fainting and even death if continued for long enough. In these cases the simple administration of a sugary food (sweet etc.), will reverse the effect.

Diabetes and Exercise

Although the mechanism is not yet known, it seems that exercise decreases the insulin requirements of the diabetic—sometimes by as much as 50%. And this can be of enormous benefit because of the possible harmful effects of long-term insulin maintenance. In some cases, adult onset diabetics who may be on insulin may even be able to give it up after starting an exercise program. Hence, exercise is *almost always* prescribed for the diabetic.

Exercise in the diabetic can also help reduce lesions in the vascular system which are characteristic of the disease. This helps explain the higher incidence of heart disease in diabetics.

Finally, aerobic exercise will help decrease obesity—a major cause of diabetes. In fact, estimates from the US indicate that about half of all diabetics in affluent societies could be 'cured' by the reversal of obesity to normal weight—and staying that way.

The main risk is *hypoglycemia* if insulin or food intake isn't regulated to cope with the changes in insulin sensitivity occurring with exercise. Food and insulin regulation should be carefully considered by a doctor or diabetics clinic before a sufferer takes up an exercise program.

In some (less common) cases of a poorly controlled diabetic, exercise may have the opposite effect to that outlined above and cause further *hyperglycemia* resulting in a ketotic coma. The signs of this are:

- A dry tongue
- Hyperventilation (long, deep, sighing breaths)
- Rapid and weak pulse
- Intense thirst and frequent urination
- Constipation, muscle cramps and altered vision.

Hyperglycemia is less common with exercise and can only be treated by an injection of insulin. If there is confusion, the subject should be treated for hypoglycemia and a doctor called immediately.

Special Exercise Needs of the Diabetic

Given careful dietary and insulin management, there's no exercise the diabetic should avoid. However, recent research suggests that insulin sensitivity is greatest in 'slow twitch' muscle fibre. Hence exercise utilising slow twitch fibres (i.e. aerobic exercise) will have the most benefit for stable management.

Under certain conditions such as exreme hot or cold weather, or where the diabetic is suffering a cold or fever, more energy will be used in exercise. The same is true in women diabetics during menstruation or pregnancy. Hence the diabetic would need to adjust by either decreasing insulin or increasing calorie intake.

As exercise increases the rate of insulin absorption in muscles, it is wise for the diabetic on insulin not to inject at an area being used most for exercise— particularly the leg. Abdominal walls or the arm can be used as the site of injection for such exercise as running etc.

Tips for the Fitness Leader

The following is advisable in prescribing exercise for diabetics:

- Check the diabetic for cardio-vascular complications which may contra-indicate exercise, i.e. high blood pressure, heart rate abnormalities etc.
- Get medical screening and advice on insulin and dietary changes necessary, beforehand.
- Have sugar or sweets such as 'life-savers' nearby in the event of a hypoglycemic reaction.
- Ensure the diabetic does not exercise alone.
- Try to see that the diabetic regulates sugar intake so that there is a mild elevation of blood sugar before exercise and a continuation afterwards (a light snack for example).
- Go for aerobic programs.

Diabetic clinics are now available in most major city hospitals. For further information, regular contact should be made with these.

Pregnancy

For most women, pregnancy is a natural event. For some male doctors, on the other hand, it's the cue for a nervous breakdown! If some of them had their way, the expectant mother would be put in hibernation for 9 months. Yet exercise physiologists point out that many women work vigorously up until the time of child-birth, with little apparent effect on the infant.

Changes During Pregnancy

The main physical changes during pregnancy with implications for exercise are:

• Increased softening of the joints due to the hormone relaxin

• Increased blood volume (by up to 30%), stepping up the need for iron in the diet

• Increase in breast size which may lead to fibrous tissue breakdown if firm support isn't provided, especially during exercise

• Increased strain on uterine ligaments as the stomach enlarges. This can be intensified by jarring activities such as jogging, causing 'stitches' or back pain.

These changes simply alter the emphasis on exercise type and intensity during pregnancy. They do not negate the need or usefulness of exercise. However, proof of the effects of exercise on both the mother and the foetus is still lacking.

Exercise and Pregnancy

For obvious and ethical reasons, research on the effects of exercise with human mothers has been difficult to conduct. Most work that has been done, though, suggests a positive benefit *within reason*.

Studies with animals, on the other hand, have shown a decrease in blood flow to the uterus during exercise large enough to prompt experts to be conservative in their recommendation about exercise during pregnancy.

One reason for this is the large inter-, as well as intra-individual differences. In fact, most medical colleges have failed to issue a positive statement on exercise during pregnancy because of the considerable differences between pregnancies.

Most experts agree that the main factors which determine appropriate training for a pregnant woman are her pre-pregnancy fitness and activity levels. Women can invariably continue their regular sport and exercise schedules during the first and second trimesters at least, although they should be aware that there is a gradual decrease in efficiency and performance during the second trimester.

For women with no previous exercise experience, more guidelines are necessary. Some of these, as spelled out in the Canadian Government document, *Fitness and Pregnancy*, are outlined below:

Tips for the Fitness Leader

• Warm-up slowly and carefully to aid joint strengthening, countering the effects of the joint-softening hormone *relaxin*.

• Concentrate on stretching—particularly in the groin, pectorals and hamstrings

• Minimise jarring exercises such as jogging. Where possible, substitute weight-bearing activities (swimming, cycling). Avoid ballistic (bouncing) movements at all times.

• Do *not* use *an*aerobic activities with pregnant women. Mild aerobic activities (e.g. walking) are best.

• Use exercises that will help strengthen (tone) the pelvic floor, abdominals, pectorals, upper back and thighs.

• Avoid exercising in hot humid conditions without good ventilation. A build-up of body temperature can be harmful to the foetus

• Avoid long periods lying on the back during the class as this can decrease the efficiency of blood flow back to the heart.

• Avoid activities that involve hyper-extension of the spine (e.g. back arching). The opposite (e.g. toe touching) should also be dispensed with.

• Avoid sitting in one spot for long periods, so that the strain on the back is minimised. When sitting, make sure the legs are bent, and that one of them is always kept on the ground during exercise.

• Avoid activities that involve a risk of falling (e.g. skiing, racquet sports, riding etc.).

• Ensure that a good supportive bra with non-elastic straps is worn at all times.

• Advise the pregnant woman to eat some form of carbohydrate 1 to 2 hours before exercising to prevent dizziness and fatigue.

• Avoid exercise sequencing which involves sudden changes in posture. This is because rapid changes in blood pressure may cause fainting.

• Teach proper breathing techniques and ensure that the breath is never held during exertion. Breathe naturally during exercise.

• From the forward bent position, always uncurl to stand in such a way that the head and shoulders are the last up. Keep knees bent and lift the trunk with the thighs, not the lower back.

• Avoid hot saunas, steam rooms and any other form of heat treatment (including sauna pants, suits etc.), even if pregnancy is only *suspected*.

• Always check with a sympathetic, exercise-oriented physician before embarking on any new type of exercise program.

• Minimise activities when on hands and knees as this can cause sag in the lower bag, and pain.

• Discontinue any exercise that causes pain or distress.

• Limit stationary aerobics (e.g. jogging on the spot etc.) to 2 minutes in order to prevent jarring. Instead, use rhythmical, comprehensive body movements.

Hypertension

Hypertension is a medical condition indicating abnormally high blood pressure. Surveys report its existence in up to 1 in 7 Australians over the age of 19.

Hypertension is known as *the symptomless disease*, because it's often the cause rather than the outcome of complications. Traditionally, it has been treated with anti-hypertensive drugs. But some side effects of these have led practitioners to look to more natural forms of treatment.

The questions for the practitioners, then, are:

1. Does exercise lower blood pressure?
2. If so, in what form should it be taken, and with what precautions, by hypertensive people?

Exercise and Hypertension

Regular aerobic exercise has been thought to help decrease blood pressure through either:

• Chronic dilation of the arteries.

• Chronic reduction in heart rate and increase in stroke volume resulting in the heart working less hard to supply blood to the working muscles.

• Reduction in body weight, which has consistently been shown to lower blood pressure.

The value of exercise in helping to relieve hypertension is not wholly clear, however a recent review of research on the subject carried out by Washington University's Doug Seals and James Hagberg, reported in the 1984 journal *Medicine and Science in Sports and Exercise*, looked at 12 studies carried out internationally over 10 years between 1973 and 1983. Of the 12, 8 showed reductions in high blood pressures following an aerobic exercise program, but the majority of these studies had methodological problems. In particular, 2 studies showed that a group of controls (i.e. those who did no exercise over the test period) also had significant decreases in blood pressure. Most of the other studies failed even to use a control group, making their findings questionable.

Given the limitations of the research, it has to be concluded that there's not enough scientific evidence yet to suggest that exercise could be substituted for medication as a treatment for hypertension.

Nevertheless, Seals and Hagberg conclude that there *is* evidence to suggest that:

• Blood pressure is decreased more easily in those with only mild (borderline) hypertension than in those with high blood pressure.

• The greater the improvement in aerobic capacity (VO_2 Max) after an exercise program, the more the expected reduction in blood pressure.

• Changes in blood pressure noticed after an extended exercise program seem to be independent of body weight (it's not known however if this is independent of changes in *fat* as distinct from *weight*).

Tips for the Fitness Leader

Although it seems from this that exercise *may* be beneficial for the hypertensive person, precautions should be taken:

• Consult a doctor before prescribing a full exercise program.

• Monitor blood pressure during a sub-maximal stress test carried out by a qualified fitness tester.

• Prescribe an exercise program which is gradual, regular and aerobic in nature.

• Avoid isometric exercises, inversion treatments and sudden changes in temperature (sauna baths to cold showers etc.) as these can increase blood pressure and put extra strain on a weak heart.

• Don't use pulse rate as a measure of exercise intensity if blood pressure medications are being used, as these can decrease pulse rate significantly.

In summary, while it appears exercise is not a panacea for hypertension, it can be a useful part of a hypertension management program if carried out properly.

16 Facts and Fallacies

A major problem of working in the field of health and fitness is knowing just who to believe. One 'expert' will say one week that coffee causes cancer, that smoking doesn't and that exercise can kill. The next week another 'expert' will say the opposite.

So how do you know who to believe?

Health is an Impure Science

The fact is that health is an impure science. Unlike in the past, conclusions can't always be based on the old system which basically stated that if a 'germ' (bacteria or virus) can be isolated and infected into another organism, that is proof enough of the cause of the disease.

Modern-day research is much more complicated. In the disease area, many of the modern ailments (e.g. heart disease, cancer) don't seem to be caused by micro-organisms, but by lifestyle.

Conclusions now are often based on probability. If several unbiased, expert studies over many years show a consistent relationship between a disease and some aspect of behaviour, scientists will begin to examine that behaviour in more detail.

For example, some 30,000 research studies carried out over 30 years have all shown a strong relationship between smoking and lung cancer. Only a small number show no relationship. Hence, although the exact mechanism of cause is not known, scientists can say with a high level of confidence (let's say 99% certainty) that smoking causes cancer.

On the other hand, it has been suggested by some that large doses of vitamin C can cure the common cold. Yet the majority of those unbiased experiments carried out to test this have failed to confirm it. Hence most scientists would have little confidence in suggesting (say 0–10% certainty) that vitamin C cures the common cold.

Of course there are always those who claim to speak with more confidence. Some do so because they genuinely believe they have more information; others because they stand to gain financially, and still others because of their personal experience. Many practitioners make judgments based on the effectiveness of their own treatments with one or only a few patients.

Yet according to the American Medical Association, about 70% of diseases are cured by time. Thus, without a careful experiment comparing 'treated' patients with those treated with a placebo (i.e. an inactive substance like water), it's impossible to know whether the treatment worked or the body healed itself.

Trends in Faddism

Understandably, many people aren't satisfied with half answers—even if that's all that is known. And when science fails to provide the answers, the public looks elsewhere—sometimes to those espousing fads and 'quack' treatments and cures.

Health faddism has a history of coinciding with declines in medical advancement. At the time of the Industrial Revolution, when all other scientific fields were moving forward, but medicine appeared to have stagnated, there was an upsurge in health fads and products—Mrs Winslow's soothing syrup, Lydia Pinkham's vegetable compound, Dr Kilmer's swamp root cure, and many others.

With the discovery of penicillin in the early part of the twentieth century, medicine regained its status. Now, with the failure of science to provide 'cures' for the lifestyle ailments of the late twentieth century, the public is again looking to alternative 'quick' solutions.

How to Know Who to Believe

So how can you pick a real expert from a quack and a potentially useful program or device from one that may be potentially harmful? The following are some guidelines:

Check if the source of information has a vested interest in a certain opinion. A scientist sponsored by a tobacco company or a fitness industry is not likely to report results that don't support his or her company.

Beware of 'secret' or 'magic' formulas or machines.

If treatments work, they don't remain secret for long. On the other hand, there has never been a successful 'magic' route to fitness or fat loss.

Examine the affiliations of the spokesperson. Is he/she backed by a large impartial academic institution or reputable organisation without vested interests?

Be sceptical of arguments using case histories from individual clients or patients. Proof of a treatment can only come from unbiased studies with large numbers.

The Case of Horace Fletcher

Horace Fletcher was an American living around the turn of the century. His story epitomises the dangers of misinterpreting information about health.

Like many health faddists of his day, Horace Fletcher had been a 98-pound weakling. He was saved from an early demise—at least according to his own estimation—by a simple streak of enlightenment.

Observing that the human being has 32 teeth, Horace surmised that this must mean that we should chew our food 32 times before swallowing. He did, and found that it aided his own ailing elimination functions.

So he set out to tell the world. 'Fletcherising', as it was known, became trendy among the health conscious of the day, with followers masticating 32 times before swallowing every mouthful. However, after some time it became obvious that this did not cure all problems. Hence Horace raised his limit for the experienced to 64 chews, then 128 and then 256.

Ultimately, he claimed food should only be chewed and then spat out. Defecation he said, was evidence that swallowing food was poisonous and should therefore not occur. Unfortunately, this last stand occurred just before Horace's untimely death, which was related to constipation and which coincided with his view that Fletcherising would now allow him to live forever.

Myths and Fallacies

Exercise Equipment

The Pure Food Act of 1908 reduced the availability of quack medicines and nostrums. But there has yet to be an equivalent Pure Exercise Act. It is still possible to sell and promote equipment and programs that have no scientific support and no established effectiveness.

A basic principle of weight reduction is that energy must be expended on the part of the individual trying to lose weight. Hence any equipment that does the exercise for the person is likely to be little more than useless. Examples of passive exercise devices are:

Rolling Machines: These wooden or metal rollers, run by an electric motor roll up and down the body part to which they are applied. They do not 'loosen' or 'break down' fat as claimed. Fat is stored energy and is only used up as fuel during aerobic activity or under conditions of reduced food intake.

Vibrating Belts, Tables, Pillows etc.: These are driven by an electric motor and jerk backwards and forwards, causing part of the body to shake. They do not break down fat, nor are they effective in weight loss. They may cause a temporary increase in local circulation and may be relaxing, but they can also be potentially harmful if used on the abdomen, especially by women during pregnancy, or while an IUD is in place. Research has shown that 15 minutes of vigorous vibration by a vibrating belt uses the equivalent of 1/23 of an ounce of fat more than if one is simply sitting at rest.

Motor Driven Cycles and Machines: Like all machines that do the work for the individual, these are not effective in weight reduction, figure improvement or development of fitness.

Electric Muscle Stimulators: When applied to a muscle, these devices cause the muscle to contract involuntarily. The amount of energy used by the muscle however is insignificant. Any weight losses which do result generally occur from the fluid losses of an accompanying diet. The devices can be dangerous in inducing heart attacks, gastrointestinal, orthopaedic, kidney and other disorders and possibly aggravate epilepsy, hernia and varicose veins.

Weighted Belts: These do have the effect of increasing the effort required to carry out a task, but this is again minimal. Such devices are uncomfortable, impractical and in certain instances may place an extra strain on certain parts of the body such as the back.

Inflated Shorts, Belts, Sauna Suits etc.: Airtight suits and rubberised garments are potentially hazardous in increasing the possibility of heat exhaustion. Any losses in body weight which do occur are simply water losses which will be quickly replaced. If one performs exercise in conjunction with such garments, the exercise (not the garment) may have beneficial effects, but this is outweighed by the potential dangers.

Figure Wrapping: Some reducing centres advertise that wrapping the body in 'magic' solutions will cause a permanent reduction in body girth. Pressure of the bandages can, at best, have a temporary shrinkage effect on cell size, but this is not likely to be permanent

and may be potentially dangerous. A similar effect can be noticed from the shrinkage of skin after a tight wristwatch is removed.

Steam or Sauna Baths: The effect of sauna and steam treatments is largely psychological, although some temporary relief from aches and pains may result from the heat. Weight losses resulting from these are generally fluid losses and are soon replaced. Heat treatments can also be dangerous for individuals with heart disease, high blood pressure or diabetes or in women who are recently pregnant. The effect is a rapid increase in resting heart rate, and a lowering of blood pressure which is immediately (and perhaps dangerously) raised when leaving the heat. Instant cooling such as jumping into a cold pool or shower can exacerbate the problem. Heat treatments should not be used within an hour of eating or while under the influence of alcohol or drugs such as anti-coagulants, stimulants, hypnotics, narcotics of tranquillisers.

Finally, there may be some problems experienced from sauna baths because of certain allergens contained in some of the redwoods in the sauna. These can cause skin, nose and throat irritations in some people.

Swirl pools: As with sauna and steam baths, swirl pools can be a relaxing form of post-exercise enjoyment. However, they have little or no effect on weight control or physical fitness. If water temperatures are kept above body temperature (i.e. 37.5 degrees C) they can lead to a build up of body heat and ultimately heat exhaustion in the individual. Also, because of high temperatures, swirl pools can be a ready source of bacterial infection which can lead to ear, eye, throat or nose irritations if chemical levels are not closely and continuously monitored.

Exercise and Weight Control Techniques

Techniques of exercise and weight control are often also misunderstood. Techniques that have been proven to be ineffective in developing fitness or promoting weight control include the following:

Massage: Whether carried out by a masseur or a mechanical device, massage is passive, requiring no effort on the part of the individual. It can help increase the circulation, prevent or loosen adhesions and induce relaxation, but it has no value in developing physical fitness or in removing adipose tissue.

Spot Reduction: 'Spot reduction' suggests that fat can be lost from specific areas of the body simply by exercising that area. Research, however, has shown that fat is reduced from fat stores all over the body as a result of exercise, not just from that area of muscle being worked.

Cellulite Reduction: Cellulite is the term given to a particular type of adipose tissue. Like other fat tissue it can only be reduced through reductions in energy input or increases in energy output. Hence, aerobic exercise plus limited calorie intake is regarded as the most effective form of treatment. No oils, lotions, rubs or other external treatments will aid in the long-term loss of cellulite.

Fad Diets: Fad diets and quick weight loss diets generally work through early losses in body fluid. This cannot be sustained however, and eventually weight is restored as the basal metabolic rate of the dieter decreases to cope with the fluid losses. In many cases this can mean an *increase* in body weight in the long term as normal eating is restored.

All successful weight loss diets work through a reduction of calorific input, regardless of the form this may take.

Fasting: Fasting is often said to 'cleanse the body of toxins', although it is rare that these toxins are identified. In effect, prolonged fasting can cause elmination of minerals, nutrients and trace elements which are vital to the normal functioning of the body.

According to a 1983 position statement on the subject released by the American College of Sports Medicine, fasting can cause 'lactic acidosis, alopecia, hypoalinanemia, oedema, anuria, hypotension, elevated serum bilirubin, nausea and vomiting, alterations in thyroxin metabolism, impaired serum triglyceride removal and production, and death'.

Rather than 'cleansing' the body of toxins, fasting is known to cause a 'reduction of blood glucose concentrations, excretion of high levels of potassium, nitrogen, sodium, calcium, magnesium and phosphate; reduction in blood volume and body fluids (which may cause fainting) and reduction of the iron binding capacity of blood serum (hence anaemia)'.

Other 'Slimming Foods': Many foods such as grapefruit, vinegar, crispbreads, diet biscuits, protein drinks, hard-boiled eggs and polyunsaturated margarine have been claimed from time to time to have special slimming properties. In fact, no food has any slimming or fat-dissolving properties. Some of the above foods may be low in kilojoules, and hence as a substitute for more energy dense foods may be beneficial. But alone, they have no special slimming properties.

Food and Exercise

Megavitamins: If a diet is balanced, with variety and good fresh fruit and vegetables, studies show there is little need for vitamin supplements particularly among athletes who are eating high quantity of food (and hence have a higher chance of getting all the needed vitamins and minerals).

Claims of vitamin deficiencies in normal people are often highly exaggerated, especially when it is considered that humans can go for from 50 to 200 days without certain vitamins before any disease from deficiency results.

Studies with swimmers runners and rowers given a variety of vitamin supplements have shown that performances do not increase significantly over those of individuals given a placebo (inactive substance). One such study, carried out by Dr Bill Webb of the Australian Sports Medicine Federation, used young, top level rowers. Blood vitamin and mineral levels were measured in those rowers who lived at home and who ate a varied and balanced meal and in those who lived away from home and who ate generally poorly, although in quantity.

The rowers with the varied diet did not have reduced vitamin levels. Those on the unbalanced diet on the other hand did, although not to the point of deficiency.

In another applied test, Australian swimming coach Don Talbot, while working in Canada, placed his own competitive swimmers on either a daily vitamin E supplement or a placebo. Neither group knew which was which. There were no differences in swimming performances over time.

Obviously, there may be real cases of vitamin deficiency among athletes as amongst sedentary people. Nutritionists generally agree though that these are rare, particularly if the food intake is varied and balanced.

Salt and the Athlete: It's long been thought that the highly active have an extra need for sodium (salt) as much of this is lost through sweat. There is also a long-standing view that salt supplements in the form of salt tablets will help prevent cramps, particularly in hot or humid conditions.

Sodium is one mineral (along with calcium, potassium, chloride etc.) that is lost from the body in sweat. Chemical analysis of sweat, however, shows that it is not lost in quantities which would be thought to be deleterious, particularly given the salt intake of most Australians. While a marathon runner may lose 15% of body fluid over the course of a 3 hour marathon, research at the University of Western Australia suggests that the loss of sodium represents only about 8%. If replacement, such as through mineral replacement drinks, is at the level of 15%, this can increase the sodium level in the bloodstream and lead to further dehydration because of the moisture-attracting properties of sodium.

Average daily salt consumption in Australia is 15 mg per head. The recommended intake established by the Commonwealth Department of Health is 5 mg per head. Dietitians claim that there is adequate salt in the Australian food supply without adding salt to it. Salt tablets should never be prescribed as routine for the active person.

There is still controversy about the role of sodium (or potassium) in preventing muscle cramp. Sodium (Na) works in combination with potassium (K) in nerve action, muscle movement and electrolyte balance and research interest has switched to the role of potassium in the prevention of cramp.

Studies at the University of Texas claim that potassium losses through extra sweat in summer have repercussions including fatigue, muscle tiredness, and nervous irritibility. This has instigated a spate of studies on potassium replacements in top athletes.

The conclusion is yet to be resolved. However, research by Australian sport scientist Dr Frank Pyke suggest that potassium losses in sweat during exercise are not serious. Other work by American exercise physiologist David Costill indicates that the body is very efficient in regulating potassium losses via the kidneys, so that excessive losses rarely occur.

A balanced diet (particularly of high potassium foods such as fruits, cereals and leafy green vegetables) should compensate for most losses. In any case, these additions to the diet will do little harm. They include the complex carbohydrates, vitamins and minerals vital for healthy performance.

Brown vs White Sugar vs Honey: Sugar is a form of energy which can provide short term benefits to the highly active. However, energy is best provided in the form of complex carbohydrates because these contain the other vitamins and minerals that constitute a good diet. The active person is fooled by thinking that sugar is a short cut to energy or that honey, brown sugar or molasses are much healthier alternatives than white sugar.

When sugar is extracted from cane it is boiled several times at high temperatures and then allowed to crystalise. The simple process of removing the sugar from the nutrients surrounding it is the argument most nutritionists use against refined (white) sugar. It provides *empty* calories, meaning that it will provide energy but little else.

Brown sugar is one step along the way to stripping the plant of its surrounding nutrients. White sugar is the end process of those steps. However, nutritionists agree that even by the time it has reached the brown sugar stage, there is little more value than in the pure white version.

Honey is made up of about 70% simple sugars, 2% sucrose and the rest water. Chemically, it works on the body in a similar way to sugar and the only way extra nutrients could be gained is for extremely large quantities to be eaten. The active person is safer replacing energy losses with a balanced high carbohydrate diet.

White Bread and Brown Bread: Although certain nutrients and fibre are lost in the processing of wheat from whole grain to refined grain as in white bread, the latter still retains much of the goodness of the original wheat.

The biggest losses occur in the removal of the bran, or outer layer of the wheat grain, and this results in some losses of vitamin B1. In some overseas countries, this means there is not enough B1 left to utilise fully the carbohydrate present in bread.

However, in Australia this is generally not so. White breads still contain sufficient nutrients to make them a valuable food even though wholegrain breads are better.

Protein and the Active Person: It used to be thought that athletes and otherwise active people need up to 120 grams of high quality protein per day to maintain their energy. Modern research has tended to refute this notion.

Protein is a necessary requirement of the body. But the old idea of the more the better, particularly where fatty meats and dairy products are concerned, is no longer accepted. As traditional sources of protein in the Australian diet are loaded with fat, too much animal protein may increase the risk of coronary heart disease.

While sportsmen requiring muscle bulk may benefit from such extra protein in their diet, this is best achieved through increases in vegetable sources (legumes, soy beans etc.) rather than the higher fat animal sources. Even so, the major energy requirement of the athlete is now regarded as very definitely carbohydrate.

Alcohol: Alcohol is a substance which is calorie dense, i.e. it is a high source of energy. Its benefit for the active person, however, is a source of controversy.

Obviously, heavy use of alcohol (regarded by the World Health Organisation as around 8 drinks a day or more) can be dangerous for both the consumer and others. The heavy drinker may be exposing him or herself to cirrhosis of the liver, alcohol dependence and possibly cancer of the larynx, oesophagus or rectum. If heavy use is combined with poor nutrition and/or exercise, as it often is, other diseases of deficiency may result.

Moderate use of alcohol, on the other hand, may even have some beneficial effects, and with the majority of the population has no major ill effects.

Some Other Common Misconceptions

Sleep and Exercise: Although it's commonly thought that exercise has a beneficial effect on human sleep, research shows that the effects of exercise on sleep are paradoxical. Exercise, it seems, may help those who are fit to sleep better, but it may even increase the level of sleeplessness in people who are unfit and otherwise inactive.

In a review of the literature on the topic carried out by Sweden's Karolinska Institute in 1981, 30 human studies and 5 animal studies were examined. The majority supported the view that exercise does improve both the length of sleep and the depth of sleep as measured by the production of delta or slow wave sleep (SWS). However, some studies showed that exercise decreases sleep in some people.

In those studies where sleep was disrupted by exercise, something like a stress effect was noticed (high heart rate during sleep, increased amount of wakefulness and more movements and arousals). This generally occurred with untrained subjects and/or as a result of heavy exercise immediately before sleeping.

Studies with human subjects are not yet fully convincing on the topic, because of methodological problems. Results from animal studies, on the other hand, are more clear-cut: non regular exercisers seem to be unsettled by exercise, whereas those who are trained seem to be more positively affected. This suggests that exercise may not improve sleep as much as lack of exercise disrupts it.

Although there has been little research on extreme exercisers (i.e. ultra-marathon runners, cyclists, etc.), reports indicate that they may also suffer sleep disruptions. This implies an inverted U-shaped relationship between exercise and sleep.

Exercise and Muscle Bulk in Females: Female sports programs were once oriented away from strength-related exercise because it was thought that these would naturally lead to muscle bulking. More recently it has become obvious through the use of weight training techniques by film stars etc. that bulking does not occur easily in women.

Muscle bulk is determined largely through the involvement of the male hormone testosterone. Although this hormone does exist in various amounts in females, it is generally not present in sufficient quantities to allow for large muscle bulking. Strength and body shaping exercises will help women decrease body fat and improve muscle tone. They are unlikely to increase muscle bulk significantly unless synthetic hormones (e.g. anabolic steroids) are used.

Strength Differentials in Men and Women: It's commonly thought that men are stronger than women and that increases in strength in women do not occur at the same rates as in men. This view has typically not accounted for differences in lean body mass (or muscle) in men and women. When this is taken into account there is good reason to believe that women may be capable of the strength rates of men (see Chapter 6).

Other indications are that strength increases in women can occur with less increase in muscle size than occurs in the average male.

Appendix I

AIRWAY: Check for free airway, remove foreign material. Place neck and jaw in correct positions.

Check pulse and breathing. Feel breath, watch for chest movement.

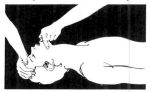
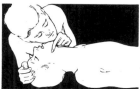

BREATHING: If not breathing, use mouth-to-mouth or mouth-to-nose ventilation. Give 5 full inflations. If ventilation not effective, use jaw lift method to open airway.

12 inflations per minute until spontaneous breathing returns.

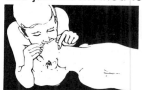
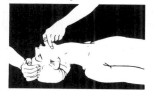

CIRCULATION: Check carotid pulse. If absent, continue ventilation and use external heart compression. Place patient flat on back on firm surface. Depress middle of lower half of breastbone 4-5 cm (1½"-2") 60 times per minute. Keep fingers off chest.

One operator: 2 inflations, 15 compressions (4 cycles per minute).

Two operators: 1 inflation, 5 compressions (12 cycles per minute).

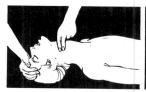
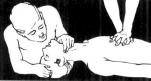

CHECK PROGRESS—If effective
• Carotid pulse felt with each compression
• Skin will become pinker.

GET HELP
In metropolitan areas, dial 000 and ask for ambulance service.

National Heart Foundation of Australia

PE.3 (rev) 1982

Appendix II—Further Reading

ALLSEN, P., HARRISON, J., and VANCE, B.: *Fitness for Life*, W.C. Brown, Dubuque, Iowa, 1976.

American College of Sports Medicine: *Guidelines for Graded Exercise Testing and Exercise Prescription*, 2nd ed., Lea and Febiger, Philadelphia, 1980.

American Consumers Association: *Rating the Exercises*, Beekman House, New York, 1981.

ASTRAND, PER-OLAF: 'Do We Need Physical Conditioning?', *Journal of Physical Education*, Special Edition, 129-136, March-April 1972.

ASTRAND, P. and RODAHL, K.: *Textbook of Work Physiology*, McGraw-Hill, New York, 1977.

BAKA, R. 'Organised Action'. Paper for F.I.T. Aerobic '88, Fitness Leader Network, 1988.

BERGER, B.: 'Facts and Fancy, Mood Alteration through Exercise', *Journal of Physical Education, Recreation and Dance*, Nov./Dec. 1982.

BROTHERHOOD, J.: 'Aspects of Nutrition in Endurance Sports', *Australian Journal of Sports Medicine*, 14(1), 1982.

BUSKIRK, E. and BASS, D.: 'Climate and exercise', in Johnson, W. and Buskirk, E.: *Science and Medicine of Exercise and Sports*, 2nd ed., Harper and Row, New York, 1974.

BUSKIRK, E. and HAYMES, E.: 'Nutritional Requirements for Women in Sport', *Women and Sport: A National Research Conference*, 1975.

CHAMPION, N. 'Is There a Lawsuit Working Out in Your Class'. *Network News*, May 1988.

CHAMPION, N. 'The Facts About Lactic Acid', *Network News*, July 1989.

CHAMPION, N., EGGER, G., and HURST, G. *The Fitness Leader's Exercise Bible*. Kangaroo Press, Sydney, 1989.

COOPER, K.: *The New Aerobics*, Bantam Books, New York, 1970.

COOPER, K.: 'Testing and Developing Cardiovascular Fitness', Special Edition, pp.130-144, Mar-April, 1972.

COPLAND, C. *Moves*. Power Books, Los Angeles, 1987.

COSTILL, D.: 'Fluids for athletic performance: why and what you should drink during prolonged exercise', *New Runners' Diet*, World Publications, Mount View, California, Aug. 1977.

COSTILL, D.L.: 'Muscle glycogen utilization during prolonged exercise on successive days', *Journal of Applied Physiology*, 31: pp.834-838, 1972.

CSIKZENTMIHALYI, M.: *Beyond Boredom and Anxiety*, Jossey-Bass, San Francisco, 1975.

DARDEN, E.: 'Strength Training for the Female Athlete', *Woman Coach*, 1:24, 25, 32, Mar-April, 1975.

DAVIDSON, S.: *Human Nutrition and Dietetics*, 6th ed., Churchill, Livingstone, Edinburgh, 1975.

DEVRIES, H.A.: *Physiology of Exercise*, William C. Brown, Dubuque, Iowa, 1974.

DEVRIES, H.A.: *Physiology of Exercise for Physical Education and Athletics*, William C. Brown, Dubuque, Iowa, 1974.

DEVRIES, H.A.: 'Evaluation of Static Stretching Procedures for Improvement of Flexibility', *Research Quarteryly*, 33, pp.222-229, 1962.

EGGER, G.: *Running High*, Sun Books, Melbourne, 1978.

EGGER, G.: *The Sport Drug*, Allen and Unwin, Sydney, 1981.

FARDY, P.S.: 'Isometric Exercise and the Cardiovascular System', *The Physician and Sports Medicine*, 9(9), pp.43-55, 1981.

FIXX, J.F.: *The Complete Book of Running*, Random House, New York, 1977.

FOX, E.L.: 'Measurement of the Maximal Alactic Capacity in Man', *Medicine and Science in Sports*, 5:66, 1973.

FOX, E.L.: *Physiological Effects of Training*, John Wiley and Sons, New York, 1979.

FOX, E.L.: *Sports Physiology*, W.B. Saunders, Philadelphia, 1979.

FOX, E.L. and MATTHEWS, D.K.: *Interval Training—Conditioning for Sports and General Fitness*, W.B. Saunders, Philadelphia, 1974.

GETCHELL, N.: *Physical Fitness a Way of Life*, John Wiley and Sons, New York, 1981.

GIBBS, R.: *Lifestyle and Coronary Heart Disease*, MacMillan Press, New York, 1979.

GRAY, L. 'Music: The Key to Great Classes'. *Network News*, October 1988.

HARRIS, A.: *Water Exercises*, New English Library, London, 1979.

HATCH, D. 'The Art of Effective Cueing'. Paper for F.I.T. Aerobic '89, Fitness Leader Network, 1989.

HAURI, P.: 'The Sleep Disorders', in *Current Concepts*, A Scope Publication, Upjohn, New York, 1982.

HIGDON, H.: *Fitness after Forty*, World Publications, California, 1977.

HIRSCH, J.: 'Adipose Cellularity in Relation to Human Obesity', *Advanced Internal Medicine*, 7:289-300, 1971.

HOLT, L.E.: *Scientific Stretching for Sport*, Dalhousie University, Halifax, 1974.

IDEA. *Aerobic Dance-Exercise Manual*. IDEA Foundation, San Diego, 1987.

JONES, A.: 'Nautilus Training Principles', *No. 1 & No. 2 Nautilus Sports Training*, Medical Ind., Florida, 1971.

KATCH, F.I. and MCARDLE, W.D.: *Nutrition Weight Control and Exercise*, Houghton Mifflin, Boston, 1981.

LEGER, L.: 'Energy Costs of Disco Dancing', *Research Quarterly for Exercise and Sport*, 53(1), p.46, 1982.

LEGWOLD, G.: 'Does Aerobic Dance Offer More Fun than Fitness?', *The Physician and Sports Medicine*, 10(9), 1982.

MANDELL, A.: 'The Second Wind', *The Psychology of Running*, Human Kinetics Publication, Illinois, 1981.

MARTIN, J.: 'Exercise Management: Shaping and Maintaining Physical Fitness', *Behavioural Medical Advances*, 4 April 1981.

MATHEWS, D.K. and FOX, E.L.: *The Physiological Basis of Physical Education and Athletics*, W.B. Saunders, Philadelphia, 1976.

MCLELLAN, T.: 'The Significance of the Aerobic and Anaerobic Threshold in Performance and Training', *Coaching Science Update*, 1980/81.

OWEN, N.: *Exercise Maintenance: Integrating Behavioural Guidelines Into Community Fitness Courses*, Paper at the 16th Convention of the Association for the Advancement of Behavioural Therapy, Los Angeles, 1982.

PYKE, F.: *Fluid Replacement*, NSW Dept of Leisure, Sport and Tourism, level 1, Coaching Accreditation Course Notes, 1982.

PYKE, F.S. (Ed.), *Towards Better Coaching*, Canberra, 1980.

SHYNE, K.: 'To Stretch or Not to Stretch', *The Physician and Sports Medicine*, 10(9), 1982.

ROBERTS, A.: *The Economic Benefits of Participation in Regular Physical Activity*, Report to the Recreation Ministers' Council of Australia, 1982.

STANTON, Rosemary, *Eating for Peak Performance*, Allen & Unwin, 1988.

STANTON, Rosemary, *The Art of Sensible Dieting*, Ellsyd Press, 1986 (reprinted 1988).

STANTON, Rosemary, *Rosemary Stanton's Complete Book of Food and Nutrition*, Simon and Schuster, 1989.

STARR, B.: 'Behind the Scenes: Anabolics and Amphetamines', *Strength and Health*, 39:54, 55, 68, 1972.

STRAUSS, R.H.: *Sports Medicine and Physiology*, W.B. Saunders, Philadelphia, 1979.

TALAG, T.: 'Residual Muscle Soreness as Influenced by Concentric, Eccentric and Static Contractions', *Research Quarterly*, 44:458–469, 1973.

The Fitness Bulletin, 5(11), Nov. 1982, Fitness Institute, Ontario, Canada.

THOMPSON, J.K.: 'Exercise and Obesity, Etiology, Physiology and Intervention', *Psychological Bulletin*, 91(1), 55–79.

VERBY, J. and VERBY, J.: *How to Talk to Doctors*, Arco Press, 1977.

WAHREN, J.: 'Glucose and Free Fatty Acid Utilization in Exercise', *Israel Journal of Medicine*, 11:551–559, 1975.

WILMORE, J.H.: 'Body composition in sport and exercise: directions for future research', *Medicine and Science in Sport and Exercise*, vol. 13, pp.21–31, 1983.

WILMORE, J.H.: 'Alterations in Strength, Body Composition and Anthropometric Measurement Consequent to a Ten Week Training Program', *Medicine and Science in Sports*, vol. 6, 1974.

Index